HEALING
through CONNECTION

for Healthcare Professionals

Stories and Wisdom from the Heart of a Diabetes Nurse

HEALING
through CONNECTION

for Healthcare Professionals

Stories and Wisdom from the Heart of a Diabetes Nurse

Beverly Thomassian

RN, MPH, CDCES, BC-ADM

Diabetes Education

*Healing through Connection for Healthcare Professionals: Stories and Wisdom from the Heart of
a Diabetes Nurse* / Beverly Thomassian

1.Non-Fiction / Self-Help for Healthcare Professionals
2.Non-Fiction / Medical / Caregiving
3.Non-Fiction / Body, Mind, & Spirit
4.Non-Fiction / Health & Healing
5.Nonfiction / Memoir
6.Non-Fiction / General

Cataloging-in-Publication Data is on file with the Library of Congress
ISBN: 979-8-9988414-4-6

10 9 8 7 6 5 4 3 2 1

Advanced Praise for
Healing through Connection

"It's not easy to capture the heart and artistry behind exceptional diabetes care, but Beverly does just that. This book is a thoughtful and timely guide for creating the healing spaces we urgently need in healthcare today."

—Susan Guzman, PhD – Diabetes Psychologist,
Director of Clinical Education, and
Co-Founder of the Behavioral Diabetes Institute.

"Beverly Thomassian is an incredible person that's had a profound impact on people with diabetes through her teaching and compassionate, person-centered care. She is so generous and authentic in sharing her life experiences and what she's learned along the way, even when it means being vulnerable. The book provides a lifetime of wisdom and left me feeling deeply curious and reflective on my own journey."

—Diana Isaacs, PharmD, CDCES, BC-ADM -
Endocrine Pharmacist at Cleveland Clinic.
2020 ADCES Diabetes Specialist of the Year

"Beverly's *Healing through Connection* feels like sitting with a wise elder who shares the kind of lessons only experience can teach. Her stories and insights remind us that true healing in diabetes care starts with compassion, listening, and heart—and becomes even more powerful when we collaborate."

—Theresa Garnero, APRN, BC-ADM, MSN, CDCES
Chief Science Officer My Diabetes Tutor

"Through masterful storytelling and personal reflection on her own life experiences, Coach Beverly gives us permission to explore our emotions and past traumas, to better understand our impact on others. By realizing how our unique experiences have shaped us, we are able to recognize the suffering of others, make meaningful human connections, healing the mind, body, and soul."

—Christine Zaveson, RN, MSN, PHN, CDCES
Emergency and Forensic Psychiatric Nurse Supervisor

"*Healing through Connection* is deeply personal and moving. Bev's lived experience forms the foundation for the empathy she's cultivated over years in the field. With honesty and authenticity, she shares moments of doubt, even after 25 years as a leader, which helps normalize fear and imposter feelings as part of the professional journey, not limitations. *Healing through Connection* is like having a wise mentor in my pocket—grounding, encouraging, and genuinely empowering."

—Sarah Hormachea MS, RD, CDCES, BC-ADM
Sarah Hormachea: Diabetes Care and Education, LLC
Owner, Contract & Consulting

To Kristapor, Robert, and Jackson-
You are my heart and my home.

You do not have to be good.
You do not have to walk on your knees
for a hundred miles through the desert repenting.
You only have to let the soft animal of your body
love what it loves.

Mary Oliver – "Wild Geese"

Contents

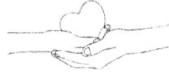

Prologue

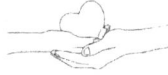

The paramedics rushed me into the emergency room. They gave report as the nurse busied herself with wrapping a blood pressure cuff around my arm and clipping a pulse oximeter to my index finger. With the sloppy arrangement of bandages around my head, I looked like a pale mummy dressed up for Halloween. The oral surgery from earlier that day caused my lips and mouth to swell, making me look like I had recently survived a brawl.

In an instant, I felt like I might pass out, and fear grabbed at my chest. I managed to croak out to the nurse, who was running back and forth between two rooms, "How would you know if I went unconscious?"

She glared at me and said, "Your blood pressure is fine." Then she sighed and peppered me with the first questions she had asked since I arrived. "Are you on drugs?"

"No."

"Do you have a mental illness?"

"No."

"Have you been drinking?" she asked.

"No, I had oral surgery…"

My attention waned as my brain drifted off to sleep. Suddenly, a loud beeping filled the room as the blood pressure alarms began to sound. The nurse shifted into fast motion, dropped the head of the gurney, and deftly jabbed me with a 16-gauge intravenous (IV) needle. She ran a liter of normal saline, full throttle, into my parched body. This nurse knew her way around trauma. She was an emergency room hotshot, adept at triage, and could probably have started that IV blindfolded and with a full bladder. But I couldn't figure out why she was so annoyed with me. Why couldn't she comfort this frightened person in her care?

As a veteran nurse and a person with a handful of chronic conditions, I have witnessed healthcare professionals with cutting-edge expertise neglect to make a connection with the very people they are working so hard to serve. I have also encountered healthcare professionals with minimal experience making an earnest effort to connect and comfort individuals in their care. As a patient who has experienced enough ER visits and hospital stays to last a lifetime, I feel a deep and persistent gratitude to those caregivers who grabbed my hand and reassured me that I would be okay.

After receiving a few bags of saline, my low blood pressure—caused by severe dehydration—stabilized, and I quickly recovered. Besides my swollen face from oral surgery and bruised ego, I felt like my old self and easily joked around with the next nurse who took over my care. But inside, I felt embarrassed and angry. I kept wondering why the first nurse had not comforted the frightened and vulnerable person in her care instead of assuming I was suffering from mental illness, using drugs, or drinking. My pride was battered. I felt as though she stood in judgment of me, with a laser-like focus on asserting her clinical skills and knowledge.

With time and reflection, I began to view this event from a more nuanced perspective. There could be other factors contributing to her seemingly indifferent approach. Perhaps her shift was ending and she was eager to return home to her family. She might be struggling with burnout, like many of our healthcare colleagues. Maybe I reminded her of a past patient who was especially needy. Alternatively, she could be living with unresolved trauma that was in search of healing.

As a caregiver, can you recognize a part of yourself in this nurse? Have you ever responded to a patient in a way that didn't match your values and intentions? Maybe you were struggling with pain in your life, and you had nothing left to give. Or it could have been that a person's fear and neediness triggered an unexpected response from you that caught you off guard. Perhaps you assumed the person in your care was drug-seeking or somehow trying to manipulate the situation without having all the facts. You're not alone if you're saying "yes" to those questions.

After 40 years as a nurse and diabetes specialist, I have responded to patients in ways that contradicted my values and intentions. I still carry a sense of regret for the times I have judged or treated others unfairly. However, the silver lining is that my missteps helped me forge a new path by recognizing where that "judgy" side of me exists and actively working to heal it. This shift to accepting people as they are and opening my heart to make meaningful connections has unexpectedly served as a healing balm to my most profound areas of pain. In return, I can be more present with people's suffering and receive them as they are at that moment.

Offering acceptance without judgment may be one of the greatest gifts you can extend as a healthcare professional—to those you care for and yourself. This action creates space for mutual healing, flowing in both directions—from healthcare professional to patient and back again.

As a healthcare professional, you bring your own life experiences, traumas, wounds, triggers, blind spots, beliefs, and inner narratives to each patient encounter. We all do. Gabor Maté, a renowned physician and author, has shared his journey of recovering from trauma through his work and personal reflections. His recovery was deeply tied to understanding the roots of his trauma, developing self-awareness, and engaging in practices that foster healing. Dr. Maté emphasizes that "trauma is not the event itself, but the wound left by the event—how the experience disrupts one's sense of self and connection to others." He believes sharing one's story and connecting with others' experiences can be a powerful way to heal.

My life story begins with the hope of living the American dream but quickly unravels with life events I did not ask for or anticipate. With a determined focus on my future, I reclaimed my life and marched forward, holding my pain inside. I figured that if I worked hard enough and finally proved myself worthy, these feelings of failure would slip away into the darkness from whence they came.

By the time I reached 50, I thought I had accomplished my goal and wrestled the inner critic to the ground. But that's when my body stopped me cold in my tracks and forced me to look deep inside to start the healing process.

This book is an emancipation from those stories not told while providing a path toward healing. I aim to share these hidden moments as a commitment to healing myself and giving YOU permission to share your story. I know I am not the only healthcare professional who has endured painful experiences and had to keep going. We all have stories of suffering and triumph, desperation and survival, grief, and reconciliation.

These lived experiences may even be what led you to enter the healthcare field in the first place.

Your Healing Journey Starts Here

At the intersection of healer and caregiver, a meeting of human experiences takes place. It's an opportunity to connect with genuine curiosity and compassion—to see the person before you without preconceived notions or judgment.

This book is both a reminder and a roadmap; an invitation to care for yourself with the same compassion you offer others. It provides a rare perspective on mutual healing. As we help others heal, we also heal ourselves. Within these pages, you'll find a toolbox for exploring your truth, tapping into your emotions, and cultivating creativity. Together, we'll explore the often-overlooked connection between your own lived experiences and those of the individuals in your care.

This book speaks directly to the heart of caregiving. It shows how, when you balance the science of medicine with the humanity of connection, every interaction becomes an opportunity for transformation, growth, and healing.

CHAPTER 1

Hope and Healing
from Early Childhood Trauma

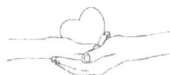

"Any movement toward wholeness begins with the acknowledgment of our own suffering and of the suffering of the world."

\- Gabor Maté, *The Myth of Normal*

Many of you, like me, have experienced intense life challenges. While our experiences, backgrounds, and the people in our lives may differ, I suspect we hold something powerful in common: a calling to care for others.

This is my story—an offering of truth, vulnerability, and resilience. In telling it, I hope it resonates with something inside of you and is a catalyst toward healing.

On my second birthday, my parents packed my brother and me into a VW Bug and drove over two thousand miles to our new home in Southern California. Ready to escape the Canadian winters, they scraped together enough money to buy a two-bedroom, white clapboard house in the San Fernando Valley. For me, the best part was behind our house. The backyard was like my own personal park. It had a row of eucalyptus trees with a lopsided treehouse that my dad threw together within weeks of our arrival. I found horny toads, lizards, and salamanders under bushes. I spent hours playing wagon train under our picnic bench that my dad painted a rusty red.

During the rare times I was inside our house, I loved looking out my bedroom window from my top bunk bed. I could see the San Gabriel Mountains and would trace the roads with my eyes to imagine where they went. At night, I would look at the moon and wonder how she always seemed to know where I was.

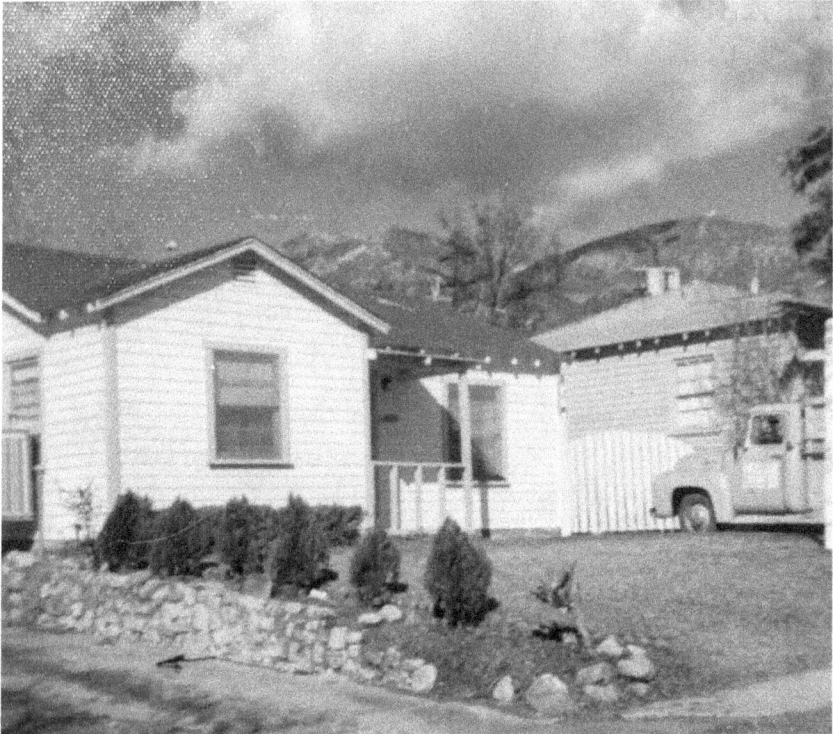

Our first home, 800 square feet with my dad's clean-up truck in the driveway – the San Gabriel Mountains rising up as my constant companion.

My dad worked at an electronics company but left his nine-to-five job after a few years because he was angry about the way they treated his Black friend. He ditched the white shirt and tie, pulled up in a powder blue Ford truck, and announced he was starting his own business: Bob's Cleanup and Hauling. Having grown up on a farm, he was no stranger to backbreaking labor and knew how to hustle. My job was to answer the phone and carefully write the names and phone numbers of potential customers.

Many of the items his customers discarded as trash became our treasures—furniture, a stack of well-worn Joni Mitchell records, cut-off blue jean shorts (which I cherished), and countless other odds and ends that found new life in our home.

My mom stayed home, raising me and my younger brother. Dad expected dinner to be on the table by 5:30 p.m., and Mom started prepping hours before to meet this deadline. I made the Kool-Aid and set the table.

My mom had a twenty-dollar budget for groceries each week—enough for milk, Cheerios, bread, bologna, ketchup, Velveeta cheese slices, and a gallon of vanilla ice cream for my dad. She meticulously maintained her movie-star figure, carefully tracking every calorie in a small, dog-eared red book she consulted religiously throughout the day. My favorite part of the afternoon was when she paused to watch her soap opera and have a cup of coffee. I would sit close by, trying to untangle the dramatic plotlines, hoping to get close to her—even for a little while.

As glamorous as this new life in California with all the palm trees seemed to our Canadian relatives, cracks began to appear in my family's foundation. One afternoon, my mom sat crying on the redwood bench beneath the elm tree in the backyard. When I came close, she looked down and turned away. She would often be in her bedroom with the door shut, and I would be left on my own. This meant that I was in charge of myself and my brother for long stretches of time.

I told my mom, "I feel lonely."

She sighed and suggested I play with the kids on the block. I was shy but desperate. I started showing up at our next-door neighbor's house, asking if Paul could play. Even though he was a year older, we became best friends over the summer when I started first grade. Paul and I scrambled up the brick wall to be tall enough to pick warm plums from his tree. His family had a color TV, and we loved watching Road Runner together or playing with his dog Charley. I would follow him to the bathroom, where he would show me how he washed his fake eye. Sometimes, he would pop it in his mouth to clean if he was too far from a faucet.

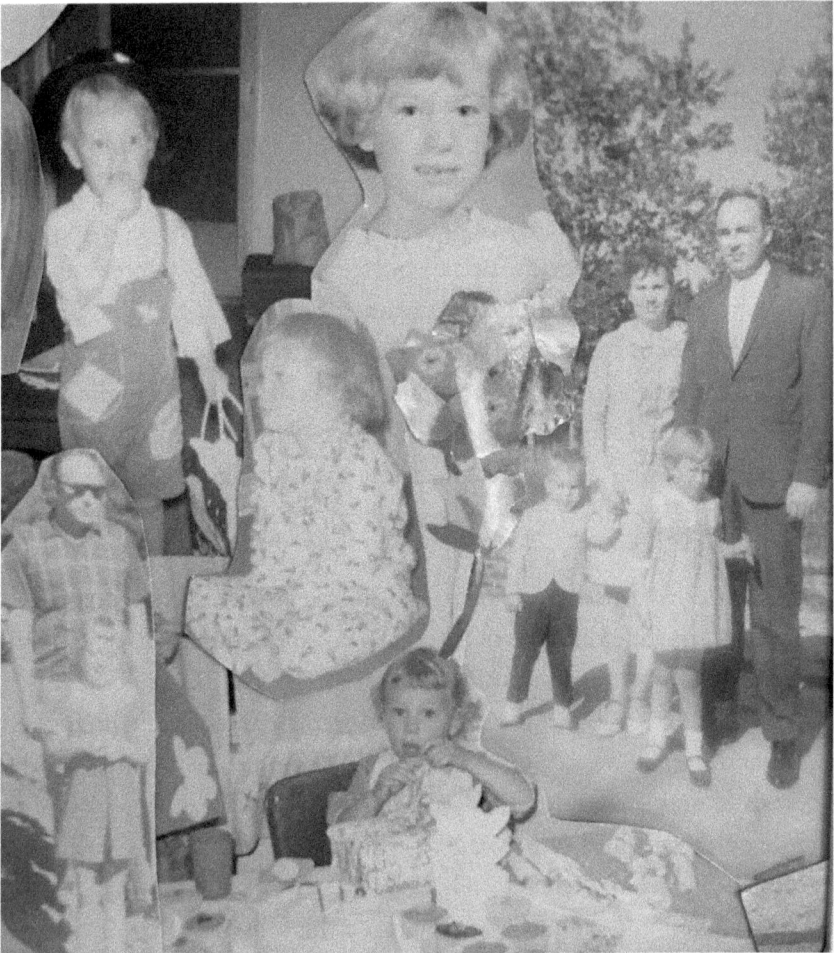

A picture collage of my early years. The family picture was taken at church.

When I heard Dad's truck pull into the driveway, I would wait for his long legs to walk through the door, hoping he wasn't too tired to wrestle. He often smelled like chainsaw oil, and his hands were rough. But I didn't care. After dinner and a shower or a bath, if he had moved a piano, he would slouch on the living room floor in his Levi's to watch our black and white TV. We never missed watching the news together. On Sunday evenings, we watched *Wild Kingdom*. By 8 o'clock, we kids were in bed.

Disaster Strikes and the Foundation Shatters

One Sunday night, when I turned eight, we got to stay up late to watch *The Wizard of Oz*. I was dazzled by the magic and terrified of the flying monkeys. I went to bed dreaming about our house being sucked into a tornado, and I woke up with my bed shaking, sure that my nightmare had become a reality.

But there were no tornadoes in Southern California. It was an earthquake. My dad ran into our room, threw back the covers, and yanked me and my brother from the bunk bed. With a kid under each arm, like two giant footballs, he ran with the finesse of a quarterback through the maze of falling books and shifting furniture. My mom ran behind us, yelling, "Bob! Bob!"

Finally, on the front lawn, even though the earth was still bucking, I felt safe. The warmth of my dad hugging me close, his skin against mine, was all I needed.

Minutes later, my mom staggered out of the house, her legs and face splattered with blood. She was holding a blanket out to my dad, screaming, "Bob, you're naked!"

We survived, but our garage had caved in, and a lightning bolt-shaped crevice ran through the house's foundation. The aftershocks terrified me, but my parents were too distracted with the cleanup to reassure us we were safe. I clung to my Ronald McDonald doll day and night, hoping it would protect me from a wall capsizing or the earth opening up.

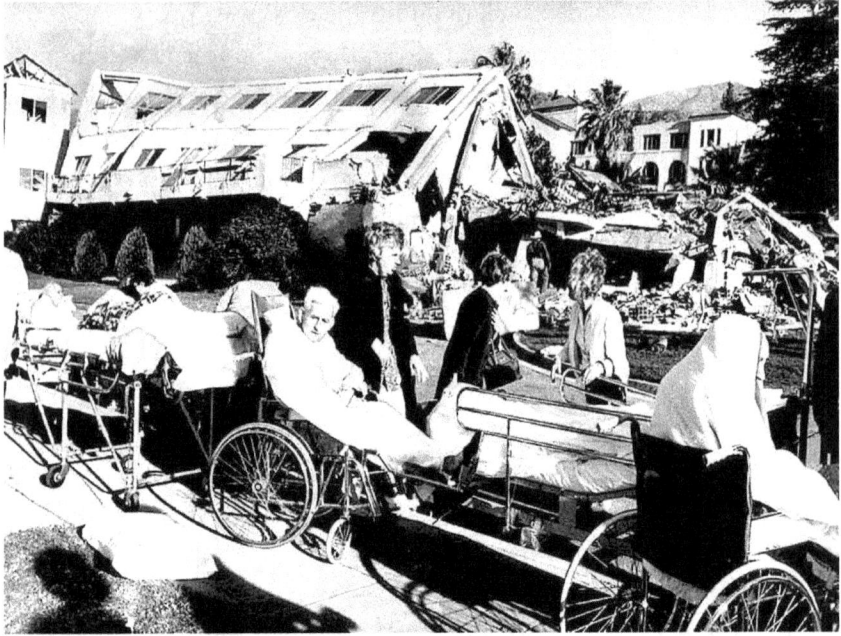

The VA hospital collapses in the Sylmar earthquake – picture ran in
the *Los Angeles Times* on Feb. 10, 1971.

We lived outside for weeks in case our damaged house
crumbled. Someone finally lent us a trailer until our home was fixed
and repaired. After a month, our foundation was restored and the
state inspectors allowed us to move back into our house. Many of
our neighbors' houses had to be demolished. Sixty-four people lost
their lives in that 1971 Sylmar 6.7 quake. A hospital and freeway
collapsed, and all the schools were temporarily closed. When I
finally returned to second grade later that year, we practiced weekly
earthquake drills, hiding under our desks to ready ourselves for the
next "big one."

In those years, my only counselors were Beverly Cleary's books
and her Ramona gang. Ramona, Beezus, and the rest of their crew
helped distract me from my fear. They comforted me as I read them,
lying safely in the grass, far away from any falling buildings.

After the earthquake, my asthma attacks kicked in. They usually showed up when I got sick or ran on days when the smog was so thick I couldn't see the mountains from our house. My lung tubes would close up, and the sing-songy wheezing would begin. On those nights, too scared to sleep alone in my room, I snuggled with my Ronald McDonald doll on the living room couch. I hoped someone would notice if I couldn't get enough air.

To open my airways, my mom boiled a large pot of water infused with Vicks VapoRub, placed a towel over my head, and coaxed me to breathe in the steam. If that didn't work, she trundled me into the car and took me to our kind-hearted pediatrician. Dr. Medler would take one look at me and know I needed an injection of epinephrine to dilate my bronchi and get the air moving again.

A Predator Enters the Scene

One evening during dinner, while I was playing with my mashed potatoes and peas, my dad announced that someone was moving into our house. He was down on his luck and needed a place to stay. A 33-year-old, charming, cocky man with a history of drinking a lot of beer arrived a few days later and made himself at home on our living room couch. He had trouble holding down jobs and did not have a long line of friends.

As a first-year junior high student, I quickly noticed that this new person in our home was interested in me. He would gaze at me while strumming his guitar and ask me questions about my day. I felt flattered. He saw me in a family where I felt invisible. He quickly and easily identified my need for attention, affirmation, and love.

One afternoon, he followed me to the laundry room, which was out in our garage, and put his arms across the door so I could not get out. He told my chubby, knock-kneed, buck-toothed, twelve-year-old self that I was pretty, intelligent, and talented. He gently brushed my hair off my cheek. I pushed him away. But he kept at it and seemed to know all the right things to say. After weeks of relentless pursuit, I fell victim to his adulation and manipulation.

Pretty soon, it was more than words and flattery. I felt trapped by his attentiveness and the threats he made. This wily predator was careful to hide his misdeeds from my parents, who provided him refuge from his previous life. But he was a wrecking ball. He didn't care who he harmed, betrayed, or broke.

After a few months, my parents caught on to his actions and put him on a plane out of our lives. When I got home from school later that day, he was gone. However, it was far from a rescue, as the situation quickly turned against me. In a nightmarish memory, my parents interrogated me and demanded to know everything that had happened. In a cruel twist, they blamed me for his misdeeds and threatened to kick me out of the house. I was grounded and only allowed to go to school and come straight home.

The deepest pain I experienced was not from this perpetrator but from my parents, who held me responsible for his actions. They barely looked at or spoke to me for that year. This incident shattered me. I felt enveloped in a blanket of shame and worthlessness. At the age of 12, I was emotionally exiled from my family. This family secret changed the trajectory of my life.

To survive, I managed to construct an emotional vault inside myself to store all the pain. My deep shame shut off parts of my body that I felt no longer deserved pleasure. I resolved to rely on myself and carve my own path forward. Digging deep within, I discovered a profound sense of self-determination and decided to take control of my life. I joined the swim team. I started sewing my own clothes, including sailor pants and a big yellow skirt with flowers for junior high prom. I started earning money babysitting to buy the things I needed without having to rely on anyone.

When high school started, I still had buck teeth and knock knees, but I was fit and focused on my future. I had carefully buried my trauma deep within, determined not to let it stand in my way.

Piecing Together Your Childhood Story

I know I'm not the only healthcare professional who has struggled with family secrets and piecing together the broken fragments of a childhood.

You have your own childhood story, one that shaped who you are today and perhaps even led to your career in healthcare. Maybe you experienced levels of emotional or physical abuse or neglect. You might have witnessed parents or family members struggling with addiction or mental illness. Perhaps your home did not feel safe, and there were times when food was scarce. Of course, it is also entirely possible that you were gifted a nurturing and supportive family environment. If so, I am grateful that was your experience.

Regardless of your personal story, it is essential to remember that many of us, as well as our colleagues who enter the healing professions, have had difficult childhoods that we often keep hidden and tucked away. Research suggests that individuals who have faced childhood adversity may develop a heightened sense of empathy or a desire to support others who are suffering. This idea is supported by studies in trauma and resilience, which suggest that personal healing from past trauma can sometimes drive a person toward helping professions as a way to process their own experiences while assisting others. However, it is helpful to recognize that the motivations for entering the healing professions are complex and multifaceted, and not everyone who enters these fields has experienced a difficult childhood.

This chapter explores the impact of adverse childhood experiences and how children can develop resilience and healing through the support of trusted adults and others who provide safety and nurturing.

Maybe things also happened to you during your childhood that you've brushed under the rug but would love to acknowledge and heal. Whatever your story is, I hope that honestly sharing painful events from my life in this chapter will open an opportunity for you to explore your childhood and view it in a new light.

Taking Account of Trauma

Your early years are incredibly formative and shape the adult you become. People often discount or minimize what happened during their childhood. They may purposely forget, or they may not take stock of how those early years impacted the person they are today. But the implications are far-reaching. Extensive research has demonstrated that children who experience trauma are at a significantly higher risk for various adverse health outcomes in adulthood. Notably, the landmark Adverse Childhood Experiences (ACE) Study found that individuals with higher ACE scores are more likely to struggle with obesity, substance addiction, depression, and suicidal tendencies.

These findings underscore the profound and lasting impact that early traumatic experiences can have on long-term health and well-being. In the Adverse Childhood Experiences (ACEs) Screening Tool, there are 10 trauma indicators.

The 10 ACE Indicators:

Abuse
1. Physical abuse
2. Emotional abuse
3. Sexual abuse

Neglect
4. Physical neglect
5. Emotional neglect

Household Challenges (Dysfunction)
6. Mental illness in the household
7. Substance use in the household
8. Domestic violence
9. Incarcerated household member
10. Parental separation or divorce

People are asked to indicate "yes" if they experienced these indicators before the age of 18 and add up their total number of yes responses for a "score." Please note that each indicator is not equally weighted, and not everyone experiences trauma the same way.

Research has consistently demonstrated that individuals who score four or more on the Adverse Childhood Experiences (ACE) questionnaire before their 18th birthday face significantly increased risks for various health issues, including heart attack, stroke, lung cancer, diabetes, mental health challenges, addiction, and suicide. The landmark ACE Study found that having an ACE score of four nearly doubles the risk of heart disease and cancer.

Furthermore, emerging studies in the field of epigenetics suggest that trauma experienced during childhood can lead to lasting changes in DNA methylation patterns, potentially altering gene expression. These epigenetic modifications may contribute to the development of various health conditions later in life.

These findings underscore the profound and lasting impact that early traumatic experiences can have on an individual's long-term health and well-being.

There is a movement to start screening all children for ACEs and toxic stress in pediatric clinics so we can support the family in recognizing the impact of these early adverse childhood events and provide interventions to disrupt these often intergenerational, child-rearing practices.

I have included the screening tool used by ACESAware.com in the reference section and encourage you to determine your score. Before we move forward, if you are taking the ACE screening for the first time and it brings up some big and painful feelings, take a moment to be present with this pain. You may want to place a hand on your heart while taking a few deep breaths. The ACE screening could impact you in several different ways. Taking this screening may lead to deep recognition of buried pain. It could inspire you to make that appointment with a counselor you have been putting off. Or it may evoke different feelings. Whatever the response, it will raise awareness of what your clients, colleagues, or friends may have endured in childhood.

Trauma can quietly disrupt your ability to heal, extend self-compassion, and form meaningful connections with those you love and those you serve. Often operating beneath the surface, it distorts the lens through which you perceive the world, shaping your responses and relationships in ways that may be easy to miss. To provide compassionate care, you need to consider the trauma experienced in your own life and reflect on how trauma may affect the people in your care. When you recognize the influence of childhood adversity—both in yourself and those you serve—you can break down barriers and create a powerful bridge of empathy, understanding, and mutual healing.

Beyond the ACE Score: Natural Disasters

Besides trauma in the home, more people than ever are being confronted by natural disasters and struggling to cope with the aftermath. The earthquake I experienced in elementary school gave me a profound awareness of the deep-rooted fear that comes with sudden, uncontrollable forces of destruction.

With the increasing occurrence of natural disasters, locally and across the globe, trauma experts remind us to consider the effects of these major disruptors on the well-being of children. Such events can be especially traumatic for children and youth as they often affect entire communities, further undermining a child's sense of security and normalcy. The sudden change and disruption resulting from a disaster can profoundly disturb a child's sense that the world is a safe, comprehensible place. Additionally, experiencing a dangerous or violent flood, storm, or earthquake is frightening even for adults, and the devastation to our familiar environments, homes, and communities can be long-lasting.

My physical reaction and sudden onset of asthma after the earthquake, combined with other painful childhood events, mirror what many other children experience. Research has established a significant association between ACE and an increased risk of developing asthma in children and adolescents. A study published in *Annals of Allergy, Asthma & Immunology* found that children exposed to even a single ACE had 28% increased odds of reported lifetime asthma compared to those without ACEs. Furthermore, exposure to five or more ACEs was associated with more than double the odds of an asthma diagnosis.

I remember my dad saying to me on a day I stayed home from school with yet another asthma attack, "I think you have these asthma attacks to get attention."

His words stung—and they still hurt now. But with time, I've realized that he may have been right. I did need attention. I needed someone to see that I was struggling, not just with my breathing, but with emotions I didn't have the words to express. Maybe my asthma was my body's way of getting the care I desperately needed.

As a healthcare professional supporting individuals across all age groups, your care becomes more impactful when you approach it with curiosity and consideration for people's lived experiences, including trauma and exposure to disasters. Physical health is not only a result of food intake and activity levels; it is directly impacted by life circumstances and exposure to family stress and environmental forces often out of the individual's control. Effective healthcare begins with recognizing that early life experiences combined with environmental and social factors are powerful predictors of future health for children and adults alike.

Taking Stock of the Supporters in Your Life

My life may have been carved out of the mountain of shame and loneliness, but that doesn't define who I am now. My traumatic experiences taught me valuable lessons about survival, my strengths, and my ability to empathize. I wouldn't be who I am today without my lived experiences.

This "other side of the coin" is often referred to as post-traumatic healing and growth. "All of us who have been broken and scarred by trauma have the chance to turn those experiences into post-traumatic wisdom," Oprah Winfrey and Dr. Bruce Perry beautifully describe in their co-authored book, *What Happened to You*. But I can't take all the credit for my ability to transcend the events of my early life and still hold onto hopefulness. I found a lifeline in a family-owned restaurant that became my second home.

Safe adults are critical in helping children who have experienced ACEs by providing stability, support, and a sense of safety. Studies show that kids who experience trauma are more likely to pull through it if they have adults in their lives who make them feel safe and heard. This certainly was the case in my life. Even though my home life had crumbled, I found a new family at a Chinese restaurant.

At the age of 14 and a half, I started working in Ying's Kitchen Chinese Restaurant. By luck or fate, I had found a refuge.

Ying's was a long rectangular restaurant in a strip mall between Kinney Shoe Store and Caruso's Italian restaurant, where you might get a glimpse of Vito Scataglia driving his Corvette if you were lucky. The ordering area was lined with a half-dozen plastic chairs where people could wait for a paper bag filled with the most delicious food in Sylmar.

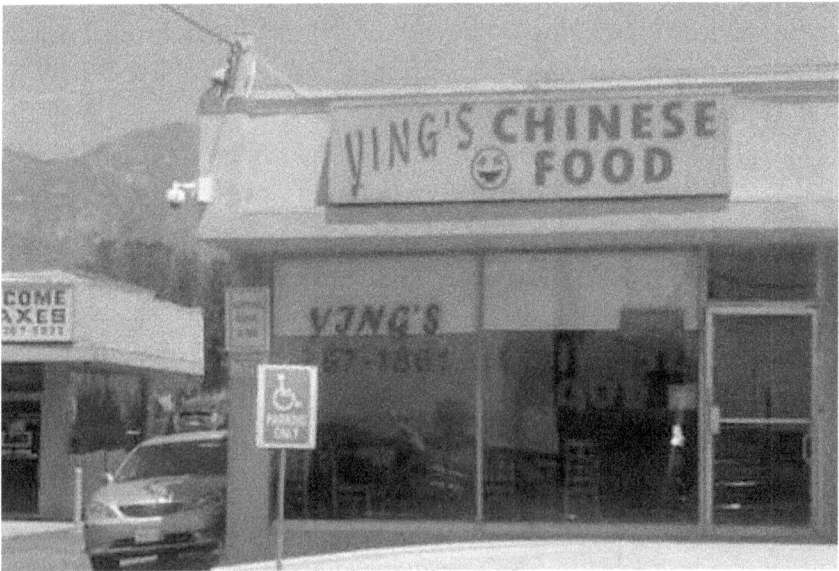

Alex and his wife, Ying, were the owners and founders of the homestyle takeout restaurant. Alex stood at his station on a wooden platform and endlessly chopped bok choy, onions, and other vegetables with the attention and precision of a maestro conducting a symphony. There were three colossal metal woks, where Alex threw celery, water chestnuts, onions, and water into hot oil that sizzled like steam trains.

Two teenage girls, including me, stood behind the 10-foot metal table, waiting for the boxes filled with chicken fried rice, beef chow mein, or sweet and sour chicken. Our job was to bag the food, making sure the combination of items was correct and matched the customer's order.

I showed up at 4:00 p.m. every day after school and on weekends. My parents didn't seem to mind my absence from the household, but they grumbled when they had to pick me up at the end of my shift. To relieve them of this hassle, I saved enough money to buy a moped and a bright yellow helmet, praying the cars would see me as I headed up the steep hill home.

As the latest in the long line of high school girls, my job was to answer phones, bag the food, ring up the orders, and answer customer questions for $1.25 an hour. Barely a teenager with no restaurant experience, I approached my assigned tasks with a combination of diligence and confusion.

On each shift, there were usually two of us girls working together. The high schooler who trained me was a bright and particular senior named Anne. She was serious about having all the new girls memorize the entire menu that had a fierce dragon near the top of the page. Each day, she drilled me on the various foods offered, including the specialty items and their prices. When no customers were waiting, I had to recite everything included in the food combinations one through five.

After a few weeks of drilling, I still wasn't as familiar as Anne thought I should be with the menu. She made it clear, in no uncertain terms, that I was "not keeping pace with the training program, and they might let me go." This awkward coaching session is seared into my brain. It pushed me into high gear, and I became determined to be the best Ying's Kitchen employee ever!

I learned that menu inside and out. I made sure to pick up the phone within the first or second ring, and I was the peppiest customer service person that place had ever seen. Pretty soon, I was calling out orders in Chinese, bagging the food effortlessly, and answering the phones while practically gliding back and forth between the counter and the metal table. Anne graduated from high school, and I started training all the new girls. Of course, I made them memorize the menu and drilled them on the contents and prices of each specialty order.

Beyond being my employers, Alex and Ying looked out for me. Alex asked me about my day at school and practiced Chinese with me. Before closing, he would ask me if I was hungry. My favorites were the pork fried rice and the egg rolls, and on special nights, he would make me moo goo gai pan. During the summer, Alex coached me on the importance of drinking hot water to cool down. He asked me about my boyfriend and made sure I was keeping up with my homework. Best of all, he always smiled when I walked through the door, showing his one gold tooth.

Ying only spoke a few words of English, but she had a way of letting me know she saw me. During springtime, she would call me over and take one strand of my hair, wrapping it carefully around a Jasmine flower from her yard. As I walked through my work shift, I could smell the scent of jasmine and know that I had a found family who treasured me.

I worked at Ying's Kitchen for eight years, from high school through college. By the time I was 16, I had saved enough money to buy a 1967 Volkswagen Fastback. My hours at Ying's covered my college tuition for nursing school and allowed me to purchase clothes, car insurance, and tickets to see Neil Young in concert. To this day, I still remember how to count to twenty in Cantonese and what food goes into combination meals one, two, three, four, and five. Anne would be proud.

When you think about trauma, take a moment to consider the protectors in your life—the surrogate parents and people who loved and treasured you, making you feel safe, seen, and heard. Alex, Ying, and all the girls I worked with were my chosen family. They fed me. They checked in with me and helped me believe that I was worthwhile. They treated me with love and respect, and I felt cherished by them. I know that without them, I would not have had the chance to become the person and businesswoman I am today.

They also taught me about the beauty of hard work. I watched Alex repeat the same task every day, but he did it with such joy and commitment that he inspired me to bring this quality to my future employment. Those eight years at Ying's Kitchen profoundly shaped how I built and now manage my company. The lessons of diligence and love became my guiding light, helping me navigate even the roughest waters and steer my ship toward calmer horizons.

As a child shaped by early trauma and family rejection, I did a lot of stupid stuff during my teenage years and into early adulthood. A particular type of man seemed to sense my low self-esteem and need for love and attention. This led to connecting with unhealthy partners and putting myself in risky situations that reinforced my belief that I was not worthy. Despite the storms I created and endured, the security of Alex and Ying anchored a deeper knowing within me, reminding me that I was worthy of love.

Considering your life experiences, is there a neighbor, colleague, parent, boss, or someone else who was there for you when you needed it most? How did they impact your life and your future self?

Post-Traumatic Healing

In a remarkable turn of events, my childhood experiences became the foundation for a life filled with purpose, compassion, and an unexpected sense of mission. The company I have built from the ground up has one central mission: to decrease the shame and blame assigned to people with diabetes and other chronic conditions. Sharing this message has not only transformed other healthcare professionals' approach to diabetes education, but it has also helped me heal my mountain of pain.

However, even though I recognized my trauma as a catalyst for healing, unresolved pain still lingered beneath the surface—pain I had yet to acknowledge or address fully. My early experience of intense shame and rejection from my parents inflicted a deep wound that showed up as an uncomfortable sensation of heat and perspiration during lectures, in my dreams, and after performances that I felt sure were substandard. Wrestling this beast has required the support of friends and family, intensive counseling, and some plant medicine, as described in a later chapter on healing.

My painful life events have been put to good use for the service of others. I am also healing as I help others release themselves from the shame that has made them feel less worthy. I firmly believe by acknowledging our trauma, we can recognize the suffering of others. This knowing creates a bridge that connects us with the people in our care, starting a healing process that can flow both ways.

How Trauma Impacts You Today

If asked to describe my childhood, the younger me would have shrugged it off and said something vague like, "Well, there was food in the house, and my parents didn't do drugs, and they were home every night. Lots of kids had way more challenging childhoods than mine."

However, my perceptions of my childhood started to shift after I suffered a stroke at 53 and four years later was admitted to a neurological ward for seizures. I discuss these health crises in more detail later in the book as I describe how I finally was forced to stop and take complete account of my life events.

By my early fifties, I mastered the skill of emotional disguise, managing to attend to my busy life despite an accumulating list of health issues. However, the arrival of seizures finally blocked my path forward. What was my body trying to tell me that my mind wasn't attending to? I was finally forced to stop and rethink the lens through which I saw my life. There had to be some underlying physical or emotional issues that could connect all these dots, wreaking havoc in my body and mind. Those events started me on a painstaking journey into the connection between my body and my life experiences.

As a hard-working professional, I didn't want anyone to know that I had dents in my armor and that behind this confident, fun, loving, and energetic CEO of a diabetes education company was a Teflon wall of dissociation. I learned to separate from the painful parts of my life so I could push forward and keep leading the charge in improving diabetes care and caring for my family.

I somehow overlooked the importance of tending to my mental health and the deep root of my pain and focused my energy outward toward managing my life and helping others heal.

If a version of this story sounds familiar to you, I'm not surprised. Many healthcare professionals enter the field because of the pain they have endured during childhood or early adulthood and are unknowingly seeking healing as they provide care and healing to others. There's very little data on this proposition, but if you ask my close friend and therapist, Katy Luallen, MFT, who is an expert in trauma with first responders, she'll tell you, "The helpers always run toward the fire."

By openly and vulnerably sharing my life experiences—how I navigated deep pain and shame to find a path to healing—I hope to inspire you to discover your own journey to wholeness. When you gently illuminate your shadow self and assure it that it's safe to emerge, you unlock the door to becoming a more authentic version of yourself. This process helps you connect more deeply with your inner workings and fosters greater empathy for the emotions of others, including those in your care, as well as your family, partners, and loved ones.

I hope this book serves as a sanctuary for your self-exploration and introspection—a chance to nurture kindness and understanding toward both your younger and current selves. Through a deeper appreciation of your path, you may be able to unlock a ripple effect of bidirectional healing and connection.

•   •   •

The adventure continues in the next chapter as I board a bus bound for a small town in Mexico, seeking an escape from the complexities of my life, only to realize that no matter how far I go, my heart always follows. Along the way, I uncover profound lessons in the wisdom, resilience, and resourcefulness of my new community, forever changing the way I see the world.

CHAPTER 2

Lessons in Listening: A Journey that Transformed My Approach to *Care*

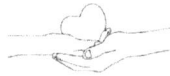

"Listening is the most important thing you can do.
It's where the real story lives."

- Unknown

By my mid-twenties, I traded the heat of the San Fernando Valley for the ocean breezes of Venice Beach, California, to work at UCLA Medical Center. Even though my personal life kept veering off course, through sheer grit, I managed to keep my professional life moving forward.

I graduated as a registered nurse and said goodbye to Ying's Kitchen the year I turned 23. Nursing school had been easier than navigating my personal life, filled with drama and a brush with death due to a ruptured ectopic pregnancy. I carried around a wounded heart from my childhood that made me feel off-balance and needy. This pain pulled me

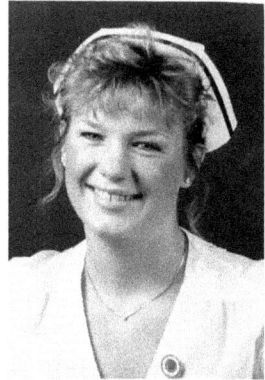

into a tangled series of unhealthy relationships, and I struggled to find friendships that felt safe and supportive.

Despite this turmoil, my nursing career was solid and satisfying. I looked forward to wearing my white uniform and nursing cap and caring for patients in our community hospital. But when my shift ended, I felt lost.

You might relate to this experience of feeling like two different versions of yourself are living in the same body and competing for the lead role. One part focused on professional advancement and the other part trying to figure out where you fit in this world. But somehow, you keep going.

With high hopes, I started my first day at UCLA on the head, neck, and urology floor, unaware of how much that decision would alter my career trajectory. I quickly realized that providing post-operative care to people who had survived disfiguring surgeries for cancer treatment or had unusual head and neck diagnoses was emotionally wrenching. I struggled to cope with the suffering and often cried during the drive home.

Midori was one of the UCLA patients who I will never forget. According to the specialist, she had "a shrinking trachea that was inoperable and would slowly close off her air supply." That evening, Midori and I walked the halls of the hospital together, dragging along her IV pole with parenteral nutrition. Stopping to gaze out the 6th-floor window to the city below, I wrapped my arm around her and put my hand on her back.

"I hope to go home and spend a few weeks with my family and friends," Midori said softly.

I held her closer.

"You know," she added, "these last two days have been the most important days of my life. I am grateful that you have helped me through them."

We stood silently next to each other and let the tears come. In the window's reflection, I saw two women: one nearing the end of her life, the other searching for her beginning. This moment of connection, stillness, and shared humanity has stayed with me. I will never forget Midori or the string of 100 paper cranes hanging from her hospital ceiling, lovingly folded by her nieces and nephews as a symbol of courage, strength, and hope. That experience moved me so deeply that I wrote a short story, "The Paper Crane," which was published in the *American Journal of Nursing* in 1989.

There were uplifting patient stories, too. The best part of working on the 6th floor was seeing the metamorphosis of people with diabetes before and after kidney transplants. Within days, their skin regained a healthy glow, and a new energy radiated from them as the transplanted kidney began clearing toxins and excess fluids from their bodies. Seeing that transformation inspired me to learn more about post-transplant care and diabetes management.

Watching this renewal sparked something in me. I realized I didn't just want to help people recover; I wanted to help them avoid suffering in the first place. I was ready to work on the other side of healthcare, where I could make a difference.

Landing In the Wrong Place to Discover the Better Path

You may have also had to land in the wrong place before finding your way to the right one, especially in your journey of personal and professional growth. My job at UCLA was a turning point. While it offered valuable clinical experience, it clarified that I was destined for a different path, focusing more on prevention, education, and person-centered care. In 1987, I was accepted into the master's program in public health at UCLA, setting the stage for the next chapter of my journey.

In the meantime, I desperately wanted a break from my current life and was ready for an adventure before diving back into school. I decided to volunteer in a clinic in rural Mexico for six months. I contacted David Werner, the author of *Where There Is No Doctor*, who had established "Proyecto Projimo" in the Mexican state of Sinaloa. He gave me the following instructions: "Fly into Mazatlán, catch a bus to the town of Ajoya, and ask for Lupe. She will rent a room to you for $6.00 a night, including breakfast." I packed a suitcase full of medical supplies and hope and boarded the plane.

Providing Care in Rural Mexico

In the winter of 1987, I stepped off a bus in the pueblo of Ajoya, Mexico. A fine layer of clay dust soon covered my feet as I walked past the plaza, where a group of young girls huddled together, talking and laughing. I approached them and asked, "¿Dónde está la casa de Lupe?"

They giggled and pointed me in the right direction.

I dragged my suitcase down the road and found Lupe's adobe house. The entrance led to a sparsely furnished sitting area featuring a built-in wall altar that hosted the Virgin de Guadalupe. Beyond that were a small dining area, a kitchen, and two modest bedrooms. Lupe welcomed me warmly and assigned me the bedroom with a queen mattress covered by a thick plastic lining. As I made my way up the two brick stairs with my suitcase, the entire family observed me with quiet curiosity.

Years before the advent of cell phones, the internet, and Wi-Fi, I quickly realized that the only way to connect with my life back in California was through an old telegraph machine tucked away in a weathered office on Main Street downtown. I felt a sudden rush of freedom. Liberated from the emotional turmoil of my life, I could finally think clearly and immerse myself in the unfolding experience of a new and unfamiliar world.

Beyond the Healthcare Professional Role: Meeting People as They Are

We all come from different lived experiences and upbringings that influence how we view the world around us. By being present and listening, we can transcend the patient-provider barrier and see each other as two unique and beautiful humans doing our best to navigate this complicated and messy thing called life. My experience with Midori in a teaching hospital in Los Angeles was a powerful example of two humans being present with each other and sharing a moment of profound connection.

As a healthcare professional, you have a unique opportunity to connect with individuals from a wide swath of different lived experiences. You don't need to hop on a plane and travel to Mexico to appreciate people from other cultures. As someone providing healthcare in a hospital, clinic, or other care setting, you experience people from all different socioeconomic backgrounds and cultures.

The people you provide care to have experienced internal and external life events that are far different from your own. Imagine how much you learn from the people in your care when you pause, listen attentively, and give space for them to share their stories with you. This intimate and profound human exchange creates a healing space for the person sharing their truth and for you, the listener.

We are all a compilation of our ancestors and lived experiences that shape our attitudes and perceptions of life. By being aware of this formation of self, you can be more attuned to the energy you bring when you meet those in your care. While listening intently, mindfully, and purposefully to others, you might recognize aspects of yourself as you connect in this shared humanity, whether in your hometown or a foreign country.

In this chapter, you will join me on a journey through Mexico, where you will witness life through a new lens of understanding to gain powerful life lessons that can reshape your approach to providing healthcare. You will be humbled by the veracity and gutsiness of the rural healthcare workers I lived with in Mexico and the people I met along the way. You will have the chance to celebrate people's wisdom about their own lives and well-being. These insights may seem obvious to you by the end of this chapter, but they were not obvious to me when I took my first steps down the path as a volunteer nurse in a Mexican pueblo.

A Cup of Tesgüino and a Lesson I'll Never Forget

With backpacks filled with vaccinations, a stethoscope, and water bottles, Rogelio and I began the four-hour hike to the remote Tarahumara village. After completing my training program to become an official "promotora de salud," I volunteered to travel to the remote outpost of Pitoreal, Chihuahua, to help Rogelio with the polio vaccination campaign.

I could understand about 75% of his quick and soft-spoken Spanish, but the other 25% remained a mystery. He rustled me awake at the break of dawn, which was a welcome relief from the cold and rickety lawn chair that I called my bed. We ate a quick breakfast of warm tortillas and cheese that a neighbor brought over and were on our way. Rogelio led us on well-worn paths that snaked through gigantic boulders—unsteady monuments ready to topple at any moment. We might as well have been walking on the moon as we traversed this region of the Sierra Madres.

Sometime before noon, a school building appeared out of nowhere. Children ran on a sandy playground dotted with patches of green. Girls wore layers of colorful skirts and bright scarves, and boys sported jeans and sweaters. Most were barefoot, but some wore tennis shoes or huaraches.

They ran to greet Rogelio but were curious and hesitant to get too close to the blonde, white nurse by his side.

Rogelio knew enough Rarámuri, the language of the Tarahumaras, to let them know that we were there to dole out their annual polio vaccinations. The mothers lined the children up, and we went down the row, squeezing drops of the vaccine under their tongues.

Rogelio explained that the dwellings scattered throughout the village were built from hard-to-find wood and tree limbs, with dirt floors and partial roofing. Sanitation was a pressing issue without running water, plumbing, or electricity. The women had to walk miles, carrying containers on their heads, to get water for drinking, bathing, and washing clothes.

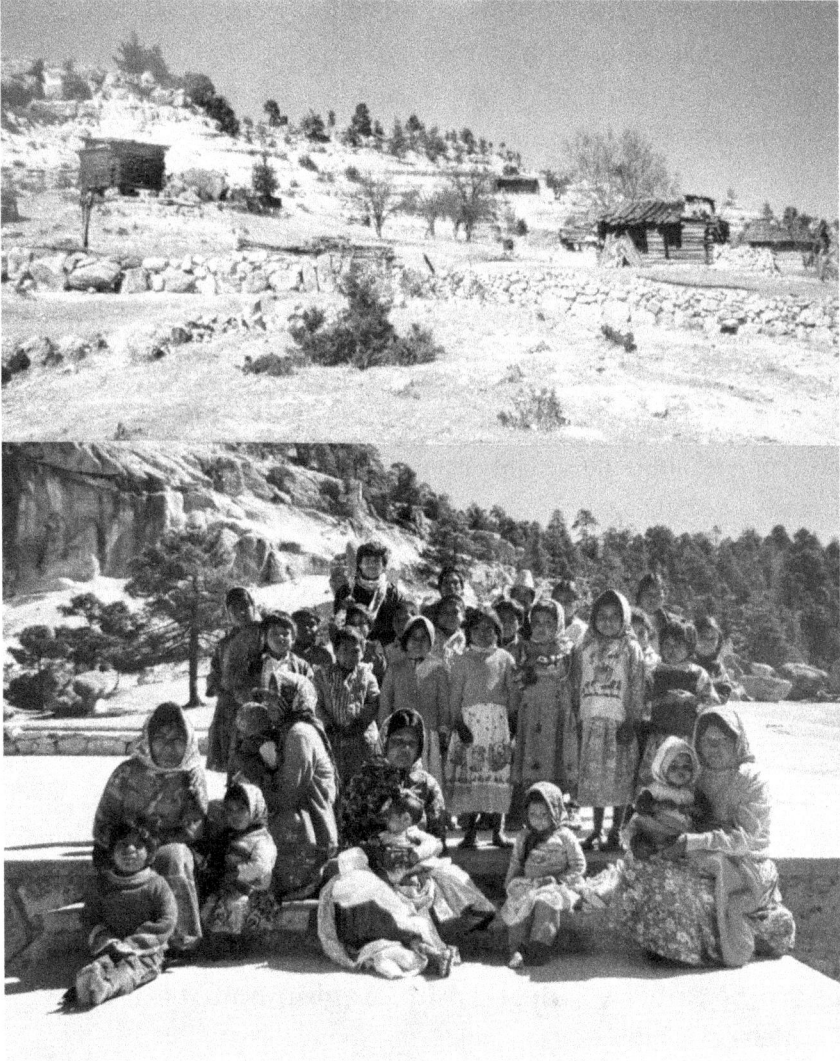

After administering the vaccines, a village elder invited us back to their pueblo to join the tesgüinadas, a Tarahumara-style beer festival. A pool-sized wooden vat of Tesgüino—a fermented drink made from sprouted corn—sat at the top of the village. A slight man with a gapped-tooth smile proudly gave us each a cup of the warm and pungent liquid, gesturing for us to follow him down the path.

We had to bend to enter a small opening to his home. We sat on a colorful mat on the floor and enjoyed a quiet moment, drinking our cups of beer. I mustered up the courage to ask him and his wife, with the help of Rogelio's translation, "If we could help you with one thing, what would that be?"

They would surely request easier access to clean water, a pump, or electricity.

But his wife replied without hesitation, "I would like cement for our floors, so everything isn't always covered in dust."

Looking back on it, this response makes sense in this barren corner of the world, covered in a red clay earth that seems to penetrate everything. Without a cement floor and little water to bathe or wash clothes, anything to improve the dust would improve health conditions and decrease the spread of the scabies that burrow under the skin, causing extreme discomfort in children and adults alike.

That moment taught me one of the most valuable lessons of my early nursing and healthcare career. The people we care for are true experts in their own lives, and only they hold the insight to determine the path toward their self-care and healing. Trust the people you care for when they tell you what they need, even if it challenges your assumptions or clinical instincts. Your role is not to fix the situation but to guide and support individuals in choosing the path that is right for them.

Learning Side by Side: Humble Beginnings of Person-Centered Care

Even though I attended classes to become a rural healthcare worker in a little schoolhouse over 30 years ago, the content I learned in a little village in Mexico is the root of my lifelong philosophy of caring for people. It sparked an approach that honors the spirit of shared learning and individual respect, and set my early foundations for person-centered care.

Most students who grew up in this pueblo could not finish high school. Instead, they had to leave school at a young age to help on the family farm or work full-time to provide basic necessities for their families. Yet, we were all eager students, excited to learn together about birthing babies, pulling teeth, treating diarrhea and worms, and resetting a dislocated shoulder.

Our classroom instructors were two brothers, one a dentist and the other a doctor who had grown up in the town. The classroom content revolved around the rural medicine gold standard guidebook, *Where There Is No Doctor*. The Hesperian Foundation has since posted a PDF of this guide in over a dozen languages on their website so people working in rural communities can access this valuable content for free.

Throughout their lessons, the instructors referenced essential messages in the book. Firstly, as promotores de salud (health promoters), we were not to talk down to the people we served. We were to consider their passed-down and common-sense knowledge about their own health and lives. Below is one of the many drawings in the book that conveys the importance of information sharing and promoting self-reliance.

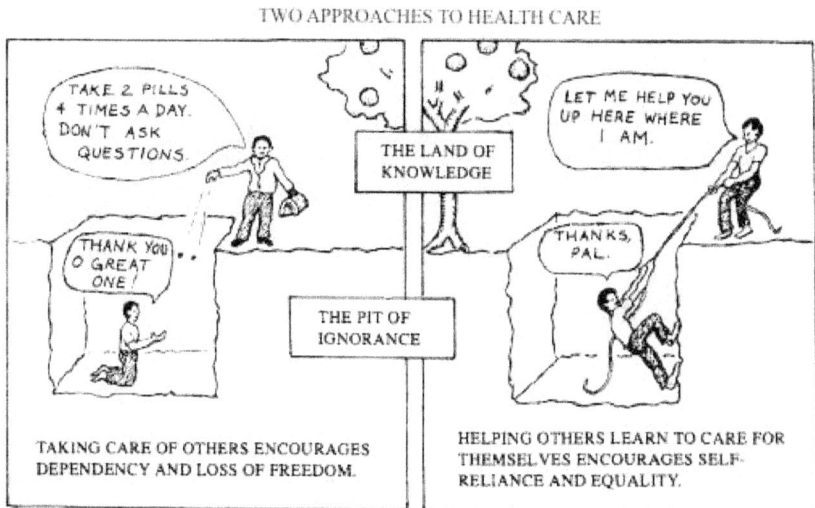

TWO APPROACHES TO HEALTH CARE

TAKE 2 PILLS 4 TIMES A DAY. DON'T ASK QUESTIONS.

THE LAND OF KNOWLEDGE

LET ME HELP YOU UP HERE WHERE I AM.

THANK YOU, O GREAT ONE!

THANKS, PAL.

THE PIT OF IGNORANCE

TAKING CARE OF OTHERS ENCOURAGES DEPENDENCY AND LOSS OF FREEDOM.

HELPING OTHERS LEARN TO CARE FOR THEMSELVES ENCOURAGES SELF-RELIANCE AND EQUALITY.

The first image on the left illustrates the compliance model, where the individual receiving treatment defers to the "all-knowing" provider and is encouraged to remain ignorant. The image on the right shows that the person receiving care is being "lifted up" by the provider to the same level. This sets the stage for a collaborative, person-centered model of healthcare, where the goal is not just treatment but mutual respect and shared decision-making.

One student mentioned that her friend's baby had an eye infection and that the mom had put a few drops of breastmilk in the eye as a treatment. She wondered if that was okay to recommend. Another student mentioned that people in her village thought they needed an antibiotic injection whenever they got a cold or flu. What should they say? The instructors encouraged us to look through the book to discover answers on our own. The drawings were so effective in conveying the messages that I can still pull them up in my mind's eye to this day.

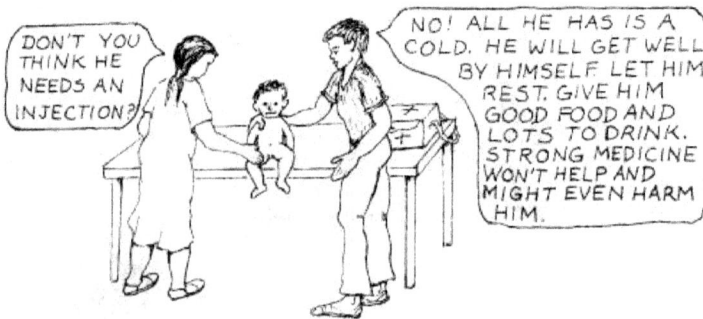

To educate people about sensible and limited use of medicines is one of the important jobs of the health worker.

This is especially true in areas where modern medicines are already in great use.

WHEN MEDICINES ARE NOT NEEDED, TAKE TIME TO EXPLAIN WHY.

The image above shows that many people will ask healthcare professionals to administer a shot of antibiotics to cure a vast array of ailments. This cartoon explains that shots are not always the best medicine and can even cause harm. In many situations, the best treatment is rest, nourishment, and liquids.

This course showed us how to help people use available resources and safe home remedies to treat common illnesses. The assumption was that the provider and the person were on equal ground, and everyone deserved respect and recognition. Before doling out health recommendations, they encouraged us to ask questions, learn about the person's living situation and resources, and discover what they had already tried. This team of instructors was already considering social determinants of health decades before it entered our medical textbooks.

Our teachers used storytelling and demonstrations to convey the lessons. Given the intermittent electricity and limited resources, there were no slides or fancy handouts. But there was a chalkboard, lots of energy, and several teaching props, including a life-sized doll that the two men used to simulate the delivery of a baby. After six months, I would return to the U.S. and its abundant healthcare resources. However, my compadres would return by foot or donkey to their farms and families without clinics or healthcare facilities. The critical information they learned today might save a neighbor's life tomorrow.

As part of my training, I was stationed with Lourdes and Margarita, two program graduates who introduced me to the community and helped me navigate daily life. In this area of the Sierra Madres, most women delivered their babies at home, usually with a neighbor's help. One rainy morning, an out-of-breath young man asked us to please help his cousin, who was having difficulty delivering her first baby. We swiftly gathered our supplies and set off on horseback, galloping through rugged terrain to reach her remote home.

Soon after we arrived, Margarita assessed that the man's cousin was in the last stages of labor. Panting and sweating, the woman begged for some pain medication, but we had none to offer. She yelled something in Spanish at Margarita that made us all chuckle. Thankfully, she delivered a healthy baby to Magarita's gentle hands within the hour. We gathered around her to celebrate this miracle and welcome a beautiful baby girl.

Later that week, we were summoned to a different town. An older woman cried in pain as she pleaded with us to pull her tooth, which had been mercilessly throbbing for months. She did not care if there was anesthesia or not; she desperately wanted that tooth out. Lourdes bravely volunteered to relieve this woman's suffering. She rummaged through her leather pouch and pulled out a pair of pliers and topical lidocaine, which she applied generously to the elder woman's gums. For over 10 minutes, Lourdes tugged and rocked that tooth back and forth until she finally held it up high in the air, jubilant with success. Her patient flashed a big smile and hugged all of us in appreciation. I've never seen anyone before, or since, so happy to get a tooth pulled.

I was volunteering with community members who had no formal training in medicine, many of whom had not finished high school. And yet, we were equals in the learning process, each bringing our wisdom, curiosity, and commitment to serve. Most importantly, we were learning to connect and communicate with each other and our patients respectfully and kindly. Unknowingly, I was receiving my earliest and most impactful training in person-centered care—one that recognized each person's unique story and strengths.

Listening and Observing Between the Lines

For the first few months, I felt pleasantly unmoored from my life in the U.S. I had many questions swirling in my head about how everything worked, but my language skills were so rudimentary that I mostly just watched and observed.

The experience of not understanding the language allowed me to embark on unexpected adventures. One afternoon, a young girl named Brisea asked me if I wanted to walk with her and her grandma to a "rosario" in a nearby town. I didn't know what "rosario" meant, but I said yes anyway. During the walk, a huge bull appeared out of the forest and chased us for a good quarter of a mile. We reunited on the road, laughing and panting, continuing on our way. When we arrived at our destination, one look at the women dressed in black and the somber faces told me all I needed to know about what "rosario" meant.

Not grasping this foreign language transformed me from my typical extroverted self into a quiet observer who could only communicate basic concepts in the language all around me. During this transition period, I gained an unexpected skill. I learned how to stop focusing only on words to understand my world. I started to carefully listen for cues in the tone of voice, to observe body language and gestures, to clear everything else from my mind and only concentrate on that one individual, a moment at a time. My intense focus allowed me to gather the data needed to understand the message. It kept me in the present and freed me from judgment or working on my response in advance.

This powerful experience is one that I still bring to the people I serve today, whether they speak English, Spanish, or another language. Like you, I am trying to listen to their stories carefully.

Some people refer to this intense observation and listening as the "third eye," "third ear," or "mindful listening." Regardless of the term, taking the time to listen instead of speak is an effective approach that opens the door for deep and meaningful connections to flow between the storyteller and the listener. In that shared space, healing doesn't only happen for the one speaking—it gently begins for the one listening, too. When you are in the quiet presence of mindful listening, both the speaker and the listener are seen, heard, and healed.

When the Teacher Becomes the Student

Have you ever been in a situation where you thought you would be the wise teacher, gifting your knowledge and wisdom to individuals with less formal training or education than you? But you ended up becoming the student in a sudden role reversal?

Well, I sure have.

After completing my promotora training, I was excited to share my expertise and knowledge with the Proyecto Projimo clinic staff. As an experienced nurse, I imagined distributing medications, helping change dressings, interpreting lab results, or taking blood pressures. Little did I know, those skills that I regarded so highly would be of no use in this clinic.

I reported for my first day, and Mari rolled up in her wheelchair to meet me. She had completed the "promotora" course years earlier and ran this clinic in close collaboration with David Werner. She was clearly "la jeffa." I introduced myself as she quickly sized me up. Since Mari couldn't pronounce my first name, she demanded to know my middle name. Then she proclaimed, "From now on, your name is Anna." This sudden switch of names was completely disorienting and made some people wonder if I was daft. They were confused as to why I was so slow to respond when they tried to get my attention by calling "Anna." There was no way to explain to them that for my entire life, everyone called me "Beverly" and that's why I wasn't responding to the Spanish version of my middle name, "Anna."

Thankfully, after a few weeks, I eased into this newly assigned first name and began to relish my recently updated identity. A month after I arrived back in the States, you could still overhear me saying, "Si, soy Anna, promotora de salud rural."

Ready to get to work in the clinic, I recognized that Mari was a no-nonsense person who was comfortable giving directions. After a few days of being assigned cleaning duties, Mari finally announced that she would permit me to help with dressing changes. The permanent patients included half a dozen men with hemi or quadriplegia, primarily resulting from gunshot wounds, that had no place else to go, given the limited resources in the Mexican Healthcare System. There were other individuals with a variety of conditions, including polio, cerebral palsy, and missing limbs, who labored in the metal workshop. They welded custom wheelchairs and metal frames for chairs to earn money to keep the clinic afloat.

Our first patient was Juan, a 43-year-old confined to his bed due to a gunshot wound that had paralyzed his body from the waist down. He lay on an egg-crate mattress, saturated with drainage from his multiple bedsores. To treat his numerous wounds, we applied a mixture of honey and sugar to his sores and retaped the gauze to his skin. This sugar-honey concoction I am holding in the photo below was remarkably bacteriostatic, and his wounds were slowly healing.

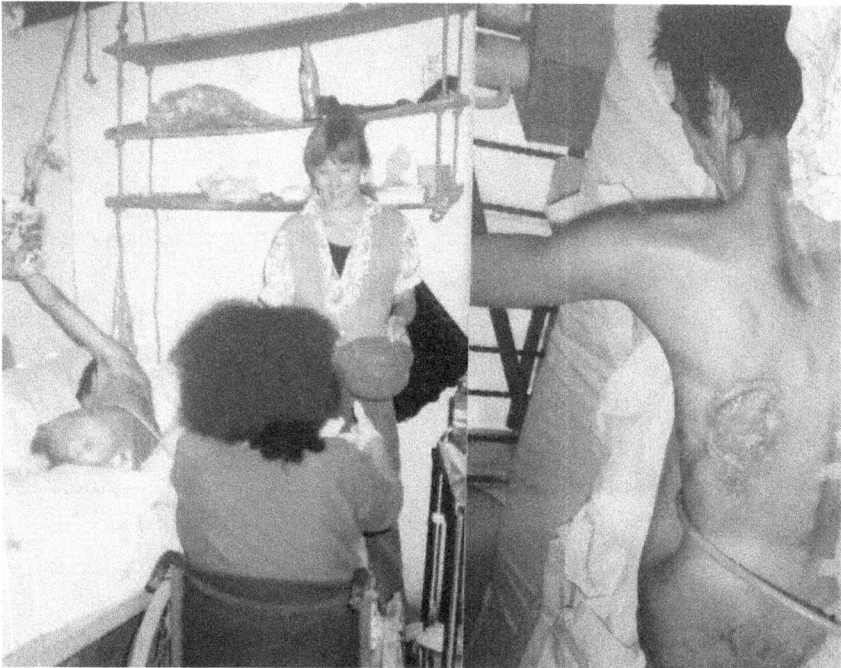

Since most people in Juan's situation would perish in the streets, he was incredibly grateful for his care at the clinic and rarely asked for anything. This approach to providing care was a far cry from the sterile wound dressings covered with antibiotic ointment that served as the gold standard in U.S. hospitals. Forget bed baths, back rubs, and daily clean linens. This was bare-bones medicine at its finest. After getting over the initial shock, I was all in and ready to help.

When starting at the clinic, I imagined myself as the wise teacher ready to gift everyone with my American-style medical knowledge and wisdom. But they had already figured out a low-cost and effective treatment for bed sores and other common conditions. This experience was a great reminder that teaching and learning are reciprocal processes, and wisdom isn't confined to formal education. It's humbling and empowering to recognize the depth of knowledge that comes from lived experience, culture, and tradition. Our egos can easily create barriers when we think "only our treatment approaches are effective." These experiences offered me the opportunity to see healthcare from a new perspective.

You may have had a similar experience during your career as a healthcare professional. A moment when your title, degree, or training took a back seat to the wisdom in front of you—whether it came from a patient, a caregiver, a community health worker, or a colleague with a completely different background.

Though these moments may catch you off guard, they are the heartbeat of person-centered care. They invite you to pause, listen, and honor the intelligence that lives in real-life experience, the kind that can't be found in textbooks or clinical algorithms. They teach you that humility is not weakness; it is the gateway to trust, partnership, and healing.

In environments with limited resources, I learned to value what humans do have: ingenuity, community, and a willingness to show up for one another. In that clinic in Mexico, I realized that healing isn't always about high-tech interventions or perfect conditions—it's about presence, creativity, and the deep human instinct to care, even in the face of scarcity.

Full Circle: Lessons Revisited in Rural America

Fast-forward thirty years to 2025. In addition to running my company, I work as a diabetes nurse in a rural Indian health services clinic, serving mostly Spanish-speaking individuals who moved here from Mexico.

They work from dawn to dusk in the rice fields and almond orchards to earn a living and improve the lives of future generations.

One of those workers was Consuelo, an immigrant with diabetes who only made it through 6th grade. When she arrived for her appointment, she could not read or write numbers but was determined to know if her blood glucose levels were in the target range. We reviewed how to use a blood glucose meter and where to read the numbers on the meter screen. After two weeks, she returned to the office and couldn't wait to show me the blood sugar numbers she had carefully transcribed on a pink Post-It note. Even though Consuelo could not interpret the significance of the numbers, she diligently copied the shapes of each number, eager to share them with me. She was beaming with pride and curious to know how her glucose levels were doing. It was a joy to recognize her effort and collaborate on the next steps to get her levels to target.

These moments reveal a deeper truth: resilience and capability are not defined by education or privilege but by the human spirit's relentless drive to learn, adapt, and contribute. Most importantly, your belief in their ability to take action to improve their health encourages them to believe in themselves. Even without a formal education, people can do amazing things with training, your gentle encouragement, and the necessary resources. Volunteering in Mexico and working in rural clinics allowed me to witness firsthand the remarkable resourcefulness and spirit of individuals, regardless of their education or background.

I invite you to consider how your perceptions of the individuals in your care shape your interactions and relationships. Do you sometimes find it challenging to step back and consider the diversity of viewpoints, customs, and knowledge that each person brings from their background? Or do you embrace the gifts of the people you serve, striving to discover ways to approach your work with a more inclusive and open-minded attitude?

Either way, there is no judgment here. This is a lifelong journey. What matters most is staying mindful of the messages you hear in your heart and head and becoming curious about where those feelings and judgments come from. Sometimes, as mentioned earlier, they stem from your own childhood experiences or past traumas. Other times, they may be shaped by the culture of your workplace. The key is to stay aware of your inner voice while honoring each individual's lived experience and believing in their abilities, no matter their background.

Forty years later, I still hold onto the lessons learned during my six-month cross-cultural experience. That experience reshaped my approach to teaching and helped me understand that listening with curiosity and humility is more impactful than showing up with all the answers.

I encourage you to see each person as someone with a rich background that shapes their worldview, decisions, and health practices. As you deepen your understanding of those in your care, you may feel more energized and hopeful at the end of your shift. You may notice that judgment is replaced with curiosity and that you are making strides in supporting improved health outcomes and a deeper sense of trust, partnership, and mutual respect. In this space, healing becomes a shared journey that uplifts both the caregiver and the person receiving care.

Leaving everything behind to venture into a rural town in Mexico was undeniably daunting. I stepped into the unknown with nothing but a suitcase full of hope, medical supplies, and a heart full of curiosity. But I've realized that sometimes the most significant leap of faith isn't crossing borders or chasing adventure—it's believing in ourselves exactly where we are.

Whether you're working in a different country or sitting in a clinic room with a patient and a Post-It note, trusting in your own wisdom and the potential in others requires a leap of faith. But that leap is often the foundation of the most meaningful care and authentic human connection.

•   •   •

The next chapter is a heartfelt tribute to anyone who has ever felt overwhelmed by fear or defined by past failures. We'll explore how self-doubt can quietly hold you back and how, with the right perspective, it can also become a powerful teacher. Through personal stories and practical insights, you'll learn how to reframe fear as a catalyst for growth and meaningful change. Because sometimes, the journey that matters most isn't the one you take across miles but the one you finally take within yourself.

CHAPTER 3

Looking Fear in the Face

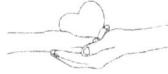

"Bravery is acknowledging your fear and doing it anyway."

— Cheryl Strayed

I arrived for my first day at Stanford Hospital wearing a lavender dress, matching purple shoes, and a crisp white lab coat with my name proudly embroidered on it. I still couldn't believe I landed this job. Three months earlier, I had been sipping coffee on a fall Saturday morning in 1993 when a job posting in the classifieds caught my eye: Stanford Medical Center seeks inpatient diabetes nurse specialist. Given my lack of experience, the odds seemed against me getting the job, but something inside urged me to apply. I felt restless after three years as a health education manager at a large HMO in Los Angeles. A tangle of management clashes and personal chaos had left me craving a fresh challenge and a new start.

Three months and two interviews later, I said an enthusiastic "yes" to Stanford's offer. Leaving my close friends behind was the hardest part, but the promise of a new beginning urged me forward. I loaded the car, packed up my cat, and drove six hours north to embark on a new chapter as a Diabetes Nurse Specialist at one of the most prestigious teaching hospitals in the country.

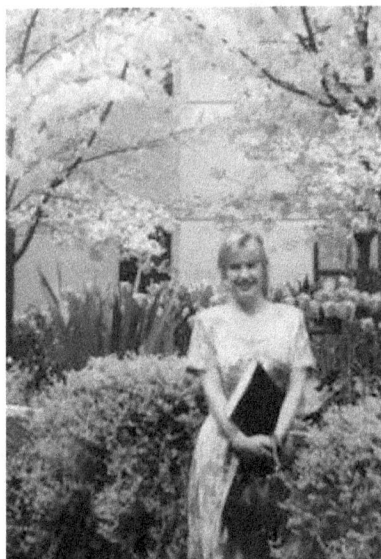

And now, standing in that lavender dress, I took a deep breath, ready to face whatever lay ahead. Walking through the hospital doors that morning, I couldn't help but be awestruck by the original art on the walls and the large, airy atrium in the center that housed a pearl-colored grand piano surrounded by lush potted plants. I turned the corner past the atrium, and my manager welcomed me to Stanford. She introduced me to my office mate and oriented me to my office, complete with two desks, a phone, a file cabinet, and a small window. She promised my computer would show up in a few weeks. I sat tall in my chair, taking it all in before placing a few photos of myself and my friends on my desk. Then, I wandered out into the nursing units to introduce myself.

Hearing that there was a new diabetes nurse in-house, an intern excitedly approached me to ask my opinion on two diabetes medications. He wanted to know if "glipizide or glyburide would be a better choice for a post-transplant patient with diabetes." It seemed like everyone at the nursing station was anticipating my wise counsel. I am sure I turned red as I stumbled to articulate a thoughtful response. The last sentence I remember saying to this young intern sounded something like, "Great question. I will look into that and get back to you."

My current self looks back at that incident with a heart full of compassion for that new diabetes nurse as she runs to her office and shuts the door, trying to hold back tears of embarrassment. I can see her rifling through the drug manual (there was no Google or internet search available in 1994), trying to figure out the best medication choice for a transplant patient. At that moment, I felt sure I didn't belong in this academic hospital, and I was sure everyone at the nursing station knew I was a fake, too. Even so, I resolved not to give up or give in to that voice of self-doubt. Instead, I made a silent pledge to read everything I could about diabetes treatment and medications, especially after organ transplants.

Feeling slightly more confident, I took a deep breath, walked down the hall, and told the intern, "I think glipizide would be the better choice since it has a shorter half-life." He smiled, said 'Thanks," and wrote the order. There was no hint of disappointment in his response, just genuine appreciation for the input.

Everyone has moments of self-doubt, especially when you are expected to be the expert with a quickly accessible best response. It's natural to second-guess yourself when put on the spot, wondering if you're offering the correct information or making the best choice.

But deep down, beneath the layers of self-doubt, I encourage you to tap into that quiet but unwavering belief that you will figure out what it will take to succeed. This inner assurance reminds you that, even in unfamiliar territory, you have the capacity to learn, adapt, and grow. This is an important consideration: confidence doesn't always come from knowing everything at the outset but from trusting your ability to acquire the skills and knowledge needed along the way. I needed to learn that lesson the hard way by looking my fear in the face.

A strange combination of fear and courage defined my mid-twenties to early thirties. In this decade, fear of failure became my constant companion and greatest motivator. Since childhood, the fear of not being good enough had shadowed me, urging me to push harder, do better, and keep proving that I was worthy of love. This fear had a particular benefit—the more doubt whispered into my ear, the more it fueled my fierce determination to prove it wrong.

This complicated relationship with fear has, at times, held me in its grip, inflicting me with intense feelings of self-doubt. Yet, paradoxically, it has also propelled me toward achievements I never thought possible. My own experiences with self-doubt and fear have sharpened my ability to recognize it in others when providing care. This recognition creates a powerful connection and allows me to hold space for their fear while reflecting back my belief in their strength and resilience.

This chapter is a tribute to everyone who's ever felt held back by fear or the sting of past failures. It's for those moments when self-doubt whispered that you weren't ready or good enough, and that voice stopped you from going after that dream job, taking that certification exam, asking for the raise you deserved, or daring to do something bold to improve patient care. You'll learn how you can reframe those feelings as fuel for growth. Through shared stories and insights, you will start to see fear not as a barrier but as a steppingstone toward greater resilience, courage, and fulfillment.

Advocating for Best Healthcare

As a healthcare professional advocating for best healthcare practices, you might feel intimidated about bringing your ideas for improvement to physicians in charge and upper management. You may worry that you aren't qualified to question how things have been done until now. But remember that you are capable and industrious. Plus, someone chose to put you in this role for a reason.

When I feel strongly about a needed practice change, and there is plenty of scientific evidence to back a recommended intervention, an approach that has helped me to muscle through self-doubt is to *focus on the message*. Remember that you are not proposing this practice change to benefit yourself; you have designed it to improve patient care. By focusing on the purpose of your message, you can get out of your own way and let the message speak for itself.

The following examples focus on improving diabetes care, but this approach can be applied to promoting the best care for any health condition.

As the manager of the Diabetes Education Recognized program at a community hospital, I had a yearly duty to present diabetes outcome data to the medical staff. I had carefully measured pre- and post-program glucose levels and other metrics that demonstrated the diabetes program was improving care. I practiced the presentation during my half-hour commute and even added some funny stories to highlight key points. Yet, fear tightened its grip as I stood before the board of expectant doctors, presenting my slides at the 7:00 a.m. medical staff meeting. Standing with the slide clicker in hand, I silently reminded myself, "Keep breathing and focus on your message of improving care for people with diabetes." I felt determined to secure approval to continue our program for another year. With the recent budget cuts at the hospital, I knew this ask would be a hard sell. But I decided this request was worth being present with my own discomfort and fear.

Looking out at the dozen physicians seated around the board table, I took a deep breath, clicked through the slides, and wrapped up with a request to continue funding. After asking me a few questions, the medical staff unanimously approved to continue the program.

In this situation, fear threatened to collapse my self-belief and block my ability to present evidence of the program's benefit. Instead, I used fear as a catalyst to create a convincing argument and be ready to answer tough questions. You can use the same strategy. Focus on the message and use the fear to help you prepare and execute a compelling, evidence-based presentation.

This may be something easier said than done. As healthcare professionals, we take an oath to advocate for the highest quality of care. However, requesting that a healthcare professional adjust an insulin regimen, refer someone to a specialist, or discuss strategies to get glucose to their goal can be scary. In addition, explaining your program's value in detail is difficult when the benefits seem obvious. Either of these situations can evoke feelings of fear or even impostor syndrome, which we will explore shortly. I want to reassure you that these feelings of anxiety are common and are more likely to be present when you are shaking things up and questioning the prevailing wisdom or suggesting a new approach. Know that this fear is instructive, but it is not in charge. Recognize it and let it pass over and through you.

Speaking of fear and putting it all on the line, I want to share the back story of the discovery of the first GLP-1 receptor agonist, exenatide, that beautifully intertwines science, curiosity, and the willingness to confront fear.

Dr. John Eng, an endocrinologist and researcher, is credited with discovering *exendin-4*, the key compound in Gila monster saliva that led to the development of exenatide (Byetta). This revolutionary diabetes medication led to the creation of a new class of medication that is now a global sensation in high demand since it not only lowers glucose but also leads to significant weight loss.

In the early 1990s, while working at the Bronx Veterans Affairs Medical Center in New York, Dr. Eng studied hormones and their role in regulating blood glucose. He became interested in the Gila monster's saliva because the lizard eats infrequently, requiring its body to tightly regulate glucose levels between meals. The Gila monster, a venomous lizard native to the southwestern United States and Mexico, doesn't seem like a likely contributor to life-saving treatments for diabetes. However, Dr. Eng identified *exendin-4* in the lizard's saliva, a peptide that mimics the human hormone GLP-1 but lasts much longer in the bloodstream, making it an excellent candidate for therapeutic use in humans.

In 2005, the FDA approved exenatide, the first GLP-1 receptor agonist. This twice-a-day injection helps lower glucose and decrease weight and opened the door to a slew of new GLP-1 agonists that only need to be injected once a week. But let's stop to consider the fear Dr. Eng faced and overcame along the way to this discovery:

> **Fear of the Unknown**: He didn't know if Gila monster saliva could be safely adapted for humans or if this strange source of medicine would even work.

Fear of Failure: The process of isolating, testing, and developing *exendin-4* was fraught with challenges. Translating a molecule from a venomous creature into a safe, effective treatment for millions required bold, relentless effort and an acute awareness that failure was a real possibility.

Fear of Judgement: The idea of deriving medicine from venom might have initially seemed far-fetched or laughable. This scientist had to push past skepticism and stay committed to his vision.

Despite initial skepticism and limited resources, Dr. Eng persevered with his research. His groundbreaking discovery eventually paved the way for the development of exenatide (Byetta), which has since transformed the landscape for treating type 2 diabetes and beyond. Dr. Eng's work earned him recognition, including the prestigious American Diabetes Association's Banting Medal for Scientific Achievement. His discovery highlights the power of curiosity, resilience, and the ability to look beyond conventional sources for innovation.

This story is a testament to believing in your vision, not giving in to self-doubt and skepticism, and persisting. There will always be doubters and individuals comfortable with the status quo who may try to block your actions or evoke feelings of self-doubt. But think of the audacity of Dr. Eng looking for a revolutionary medicine in the saliva of a venomous lizard and be reassured that greatness starts with an idea. Acknowledge the doubters with a wink and a nod and keep moving forward.

Apply for the Job You Are Not Qualified for and Learn to Manage Up

The job at Stanford was not the first one I felt unqualified to apply for. Fresh from graduating from UCLA with a master's degree in public health, I landed a job as the manager of the Health Education Department at a health maintenance organization in Los Angeles.

Even though I completely lacked managerial experience, the person interviewing me immediately recognized my enthusiasm, optimism, and work ethic. My soon-to-be boss was a female trailblazer in the organization, and she believed in promoting women.

In this new role, I led a team of seven health education specialists across more than 20 clinics in Southern California, providing individual counseling and group classes on chronic disease management, including diabetes. It was my first experience supervising healthcare professionals—all older than me.

To succeed, I quickly recognized that I needed to master two things: effective management and expanding my knowledge to confidently teach classes on various health topics, from asthma and pregnancy to weight management and diabetes. The learning curve was steep, but I was determined to meet the challenge head-on.

I was lucky to work with a very independent group of health education professionals who appreciated my hands-off and encouraging management style. However, my new boss was a different story. She left me endless voice messages filled with new assignments and projects that I didn't consent to or discuss with her. No wonder she was attracted to my work ethic and youth; she recognized that I would have the energy to keep up with her demands and strive to succeed.

After two years of trying to meet her unrealistic expectations, I began implementing the essential skill of managing up. At our annual review, even though I was scared to death, I politely asked if I could give her some feedback on her management approach. She blinked her eyes in surprise but was kind enough to listen to my feedback. I cautiously outlined a few strategies to improve our working relationship, including involving me in decision-making before assigning me new projects.

When I left that job two years later to work at Stanford, she thanked me for speaking up and being honest. Even though I was terrified of sharing my honest feedback at the time, my boss's response taught me that speaking up with kindness and integrity on your behalf can improve your work life and even create a more authentic connection.

Getting Out of Your Comfort Zone

Starting a new job or project can feel overwhelming as you navigate the many responsibilities and expectations that come with it. But I want to encourage you to say yes to opportunities that push you beyond your comfort zone. Even when it feels intimidating, embracing new challenges can unlock unexpected growth.

I had a lot of growing to do in this early career position as a manager and health educator. Besides taking a crash course on management, I needed to get up to speed on learning about chronic disease management. Until then, I had spent my professional life as a floor nurse in the hospital setting, teaching patients at the bedside. This new job required me to learn a curriculum of unfamiliar content, stand in front of our HMO members, and lecture on health topics I knew little about. I practically memorized the detailed curriculum, so I would be ready to teach the next group of members about their health conditions, ranging from asthma to preparing for labor and delivery.

The two scariest topics for me were pregnancy and diabetes since those were the areas I knew the least about. I was sure the attendees and my staff could detect my unease and fear, but I kept practicing and trying new teaching approaches. After a year, I felt more confident in the content and was developing my own teaching swag. After three years of teaching, my initial fear had transformed into excitement. I loved sharing health information and kept trying new approaches to make the content relevant and engaging. I also passed my diabetes educator exam and gained a new title, Certified Diabetes Educator (CDE).

You never know what skills you're acquiring for your future self. Looking back, it's almost amusing to think that those countless hours spent memorizing curriculum, teaching in front of groups, and earning my diabetes certification were quietly laying the foundation for my journey as a professional speaker and diabetes nurse specialist. Dive into the challenges before you, knowing you are gaining valuable skills and knowledge to benefit your future self.

As you consider your future life, I encourage you to say "yes" more than "no." Take the risk, apply for that position you don't feel qualified for, sign up for the exam, and step out of your comfort zone to pursue your dreams. I am not saying it won't be scary; it could be terrifying. Take a deep breath, close your eyes, and imagine that step forward. I believe in you.

As Mark Twain suggests, "Twenty years from now, you will be more disappointed by the things you didn't do than the ones you did do. So, throw off the bowlines. Sail away from the safe harbor. Catch the trade winds in your sails. Explore. Dream. Discover."

Recognizing Impostor Syndrome

We have discussed the fear of taking risks, but have you experienced fear or self-doubt about your intellect, skills, or accomplishments, even though your success is evident to everyone? Fear and self-doubt can go hand in hand with impostor syndrome. This common syndrome affects up to half of high-achieving women in male-dominated industries. However, men also experience impostor syndrome, although they may be less likely to admit it or seek help.

Even after running my company for over 25 years, I still experience moments of doubt, feeling as if I've somehow faked my way to where I am. At times, someone might pull back the curtain and expose me as just a kid from Sylmar, trying to prove myself while holding everything together. From my first post-graduate job as a Health Education Department manager at 28 to becoming a CEO, I've wrestled with the fear of being seen as an impostor—not smart enough, not qualified enough, not experienced enough. These feelings stem from deep-rooted childhood self-doubt and the real possibility of failing.

The truth is, I've made mistakes, plenty of them. I've stumbled, I've messed up, and yes, I've even failed. But I am not a failure.

Anyone who takes that first shaky step forward, who dares to raise a hand in defiance of fear, has already won a quiet victory. Like many of you, I still wrestle with impostor syndrome. But when it was time to step into the next chapter of my life, I pulled on my big girl pants, took a deep breath, and chose courage over fear.

Proving Your Worth and the "Stanford Way"

Have you ever been so flattered to be offered your dream job that you forgot to ask detailed questions that might be kind of important? Like, how will you be evaluated? Or maybe the employer was so thrilled to have you join the team that they forgot to mention specific responsibilities that would determine whether or not you can keep your job.

I sure have.

There was one minor detail about my position at Stanford that no one described in the job interview, but I quickly realized I had better buckle up and step on the throttle. A week into my new role, the Stanford Nursing research team called me to their office to inform me that I had one year to demonstrate that I could save the hospital as much money as my annual salary. My charge was to save $60,000 a year by reducing the length of stay for people with diabetes and preventing re-admission for diabetes hyperglycemic crises. Even though I left the researcher's office smiling, this conversation activated one hell of a fear response. I didn't realize my job security hinged on proving my worth within the year. This fear activated an intensive focus on determining the most urgent diabetes issues in the hospital and then identifying solutions to fix them.

But first, I needed to figure out the lay of the land. It soon became evident that to move forward, I would need to adopt the "Stanford way." That was code for working long hours, volunteering for extra duties, and running my butt off. I wore a beeper that never seemed to quiet down. Interns, residents, and nurses contacted me to help manage very sick people with elevated blood glucose levels due to infections, pancreatitis, new diagnoses, steroids, organ transplants, and more. Since I was the only diabetes nurse for the 500-bed hospital, I ran up and down those four flights of stairs countless times a day, adjusting insulin doses, training staff, sitting next to patients, and carefully listening to their stories.

I studied my big Joslin diabetes textbook at night and tried to memorize each word I read and nail down the complicated pathophysiology of diabetes. Attempting to outpace my impostor syndrome by expanding my clinical knowledge was exhausting but thrilling. I was determined not to fail and to prove I was worthy of this position. I said yes to everything to gain as much hands-on experience as possible. As my clinical confidence grew, my fear started to quiet.

In the clinical setting, I was making significant strides in learning about managing patients with diabetes complicated by a wide variety of other conditions, including cancer, organ transplants, heart disease, kidney failure, and many others. Through careful listening, being curious, looking at labs, and reading articles, I started recognizing patterns in blood glucose trends and similarities in different patient situations. I began to understand which hospital systems were effective in providing diabetes care and where the gaps were.

After a month of investigation, I had a plan and was ready to move forward. I was excited to present my ideas to the research team, knowing that this intervention would ultimately improve the care that people with diabetes receive, regardless of whether or not I saved the hospital enough money to secure my position.

Measuring Success

When asked to demonstrate your worth in a new position, it's tempting to dive in and immediately start fixing things. However, if the situation allows, hold back for a little while. Take time to gather baseline data first. This ensures that you can measure the impact of any changes you implement and demonstrate the positive results of your actions. Your intervention might result in fewer complications, improved glucose levels, increased patient or provider satisfaction, or fewer emergency room visits. By measuring and quantifying your efforts, you can objectively assess your success or pinpoint areas for system improvement.

Quantifying your work isn't only about numbers; it's about ensuring that your intentions lead to meaningful outcomes, giving insight into what works, what doesn't, and where your team and organization can grow. It also lets the management team know you are making valuable contributions and demonstrating your worth.

Through my preliminary hospital investigation, I discovered two facts. First, blood glucose levels were often greater than 250 mg/dL, which was significantly above the desired glucose targets. Second, elevated blood glucose levels delayed discharge and increased risk of unnecessary complications. Insurance companies imposed fixed reimbursement rates based on diagnosis and expected length of stay. Extended hospital stays resulted in lost hospital revenue. These elevated blood glucose levels resulted from not having a standardized insulin management plan. Each intern dutifully followed their attending doctor's approach. We needed to collect baseline data on glucose levels in the hospital to better understand the extent of hyperglycemia and verify root causes.

To fully investigate this issue and drive meaningful improvements, we recognized the need to expand our efforts through a collaborative approach. We identified a nurse representative from each unit and established a Diabetes Resource Committee pictured on the next page. This dedicated team played a critical role in conducting chart audits, reviewing thousands of pre-and post-glucose results to inform our quality improvement strategies.

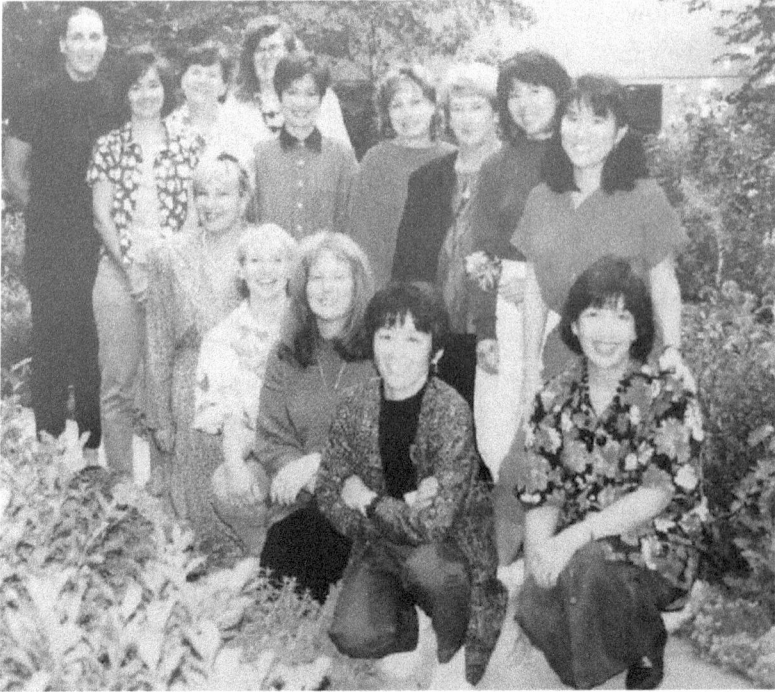

Diabetes Resource Committee at Stanford Hospital

Then, we collaborated with Richard Caldwell and the pharmacy department to develop a standardized approach to insulin management based on the patient's presentation. We printed these standardized insulin scales on laminated pocketcards as pictured on next page. The physicians and hospital staff went wild with appreciation. They immediately started using these scales, thrilled to finally have a simple, fast, and practical approach to insulin management of glucose levels.

After gathering glucose data, we measured inpatient glucose levels and tracked the length of stay. As glucose levels improved, the length of stay shortened. The research team and upper management were thrilled with our approach and the results. Improving glucose levels through a standardized insulin scale improved outcomes, decreased length of stay, increased physician satisfaction, and saved way more money than my annual salary. Plus, I got to keep my job.

Regular Insulin Sliding Scale   🛡 Stanford Health Services

Goal: To maintain glucose between **70 - 200**. This scale should be
used for no more than two days as the **only** method of glucose control.

Regular Insulin Sliding Scale Before Meals				Night (HS) Sliding Scale to prevent AM hypoglycemia	
Blood Sugar	Mild thin, NPO, or elderly	Moderate Avg. wt & eating	Aggressive On steroids or infected	Blood Sugar	Treat-ment
< 60 (4 oz OJ or 1amp D50. Check glucose in 15 mins) Call HO				< 60 see left	
60 - 150	no insulin	no insulin	no insulin	60 - 150	no insulin
150 - 200	no insulin	3 units	4 units	150 - 200	no insulin
201 - 250	2 units	5 units	6 units	201 - 250	2 units
251 - 300	4 units	7 units	10 units	251 - 300	3 units
301 - 350	6 units	9 units	12 units	301 - 350	4 units
351 - 400	8 units	11 units	15 units	351 - 400	5 units
> 400 call HO.				>400 call HO	

1/97

You are Enough

Before I move on, I want to make an important observation. We
accomplished this win without the support of our endocrinology team
or a lead physician. Our success was due to a nursing/pharmacy collaboration combined with data to demonstrate an effective solution to
a long-standing problem. We focused on three fundamental principles:
simplicity, teamwork, and decreasing barriers to move this project forward. The staff loved the simplicity of the insulin scale printed on a
pocket card and automated in the pharmacy, so the medical team no
longer had to write out the insulin plan in longhand. By aligning with
the pharmacy department, we quickly achieved pharmacy and therapeutic committee approval, and insulin errors throughout the hospital
decreased. We did run into some small roadblocks, but we promptly
addressed those and devised winning solutions.

I presented this PocketCard approach to insulin management
at the national ADCES diabetes meeting in 1996 to a packed room
of three hundred diabetes educators battling the same issue at their

hospitals. Within the next five years, most hospitals across the country adopted this novel approach to insulin management that was dreamed up by a young diabetes nurse whose chose not to let her fear derail her dreams. Her willingness to believe in herself and initiate a movement did more than demonstrate her value at Stanford Hospital; it affirmed her capacity to think big and enact bold changes.

You may sometimes think you are not enough. You may doubt your ability to envision change and take action. You may feel that you need a physician leader at the helm. However, while interdisciplinary consideration is desirable, sometimes a smaller group of worker bees with more dedicated time is best positioned to take the lead role.

Take a moment to consider if you have backed away from an initiative or project due to your fear of not being enough. Then, reconsider that project and envision the steps needed to make it happen. Just like the ordinary folks of Mexico fighting their way to better health, I believe in your vision to improve the quality of care and enact change. Like Brene Brown famously says, "You are enough." And as my literary consultant and publishing coach Joylynn M. Ross says, "You are actually *more* than enough." So, give fear a swift kick and watch it float over the horizon. Stand tall in your own brilliance and take that first bold step forward.

The Emotional Impact of Diabetes Care

While finding ways to lower hospital costs of diabetes care was a key part of my job, I had plenty of other responsibilities. I was, first and foremost, a nurse, and my priority was to provide care to patients who were battling a scary and often debilitating illness.

When I first started meeting with patients at Stanford, I was so focused on making sure that I got all the diabetes pathophysiology, medications, and labs right that I often felt fearful acknowledging the big emotions in the room as I listened to people with diabetes share their stories and grapple with the impact it had of their lives. Looking back, I realized that I was scared of the fear I saw reflected in my patients' faces. I wanted to run away from the intense feelings that the patients' pain evoked in me. I wanted to be able to fix their suffering and make things better. Instead of being present with the pain, I often switched to cheerleader mode. I enthusiastically painted a shiny picture of their situation, not realizing how unhelpful this was for patients who did not fully understand or know what to do with their fear.

A special young lady who received a double lung transplant due to cystic fibrosis is still vivid in my memory. Her elevated blood glucose levels reflected a transplanted organ in trouble. I would stop in her isolation room on most days to check in on her physical and emotional health. We discovered we were born on the same day, a few years apart. She would look at me hungrily and ask me about my life as I calculated out insulin dosing to get her blood glucose back on target.

One day, as I was about to leave her room, she asked me if she was dying. I tried to reassure her and told her, "You are a fighter, and, of course, you will make it." But my words felt hollow, and I left her room feeling defeated. Tragically, the transplant didn't work, and Dottie never made it out of the hospital. Somehow, it felt like I had let her down. I wonder how the older version of myself would have handled that intense moment my younger self was unprepared for. I still think of Dottie thirty years later, especially when hiking by the ocean. I take a deep breath of cool, clean air, expanding my lungs, imagining her with me.

Being a healthcare professional means you get to allow room for people to express the complexity of their feelings. Diabetes management is not only about managing glucose levels or knowing medication protocols; it's deeply personal for each individual. When you make room for people's emotions, you're addressing a part of their experience that often goes unspoken yet is essential for healing and self-care. Being present and validating their feelings shows those in your care that they're seen and heard, which can be incredibly comforting and empowering. Taking this human-centered approach creates an important connection that encourages individuals to keep moving forward in their care.

Standing with Fear

Most days, I feel energized and confident, ready to run a company, lecture to large audiences, and make clinical recommendations. Some days, though, fear and self-doubt show up and give me a run for my money. With time and counseling, I have tried to look at fear as a companion that urges me forward to always do my best.

Now, I try to acknowledge my fear with a casual greeting and question. "Hello, fear! What are you trying to tell me?" Sometimes, this direct inquiry will tell me why it arrived and suggest an action. Sometimes, though, fear is stubborn and refuses to take leave. Occasionally, when I lecture to large groups, I can feel my heart pound and my palms sweat, but I choose to stand with my fear and move forward. I whisper to my fear, "I am okay and good enough." I get back in my body, breathe, and find a friendly face in the audience who I know is cheering me on. And I keep going.

The truth is, fear isn't going anywhere. It's part of me, just as it's part of you. The trick is learning when to listen to it and when to silence it. With each small victory, its power diminishes, leaving room for you to take the lead. I encourage you to trust yourself, no matter how scary, and dive into your life with the ferocity it deserves.

• • •

In the next chapter, I will cheer you on as you take that leap and step into your possibilities. It's time to embrace your dream, design an innovative program, or finally pitch that idea to your boss. Pursuing the "thing" you've been dreaming about might feel terrifying, exhilarating, or a little bit of both. All feelings are welcome here. So go ahead—turn the page and let's see what unfolds.

CHAPTER 4

Daring to Dream

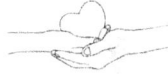

"For there is always light, if only we're brave enough to see it.
If only we're brave enough to be it."

- Amanda Gorman

When I turned 30, I made a list of dreams and aspirations for my future. It included the typical things: living closer to nature, getting married, working as a nurse, and going backpacking. Nowhere on that list, however, was "marry a younger pharmacist and start your own company." And yet, here I was, standing at the edge of an unexpected new chapter—and I felt lost.

After working at Stanford for three years, an enthusiastic and sincere pharmacy student stopped me in the hall and introduced himself with a big smile. "Hi, I'm Kris Thomassian. Would you mind if I shadowed you for a few hours to learn more about diabetes?"

"Sure," I replied. I then reached out, grabbed his tie, and said, "Nice tie." The rest is history. Two years later, we were engaged and then married.

Choosing this relationship meant letting go of the career I worked hard to build and embracing something entirely new. It was scary, but

I listened to my heart and took the leap. At 35, I left my dream job at Stanford and moved to a rural town in Northern California where Kris was launching his pharmacy career.

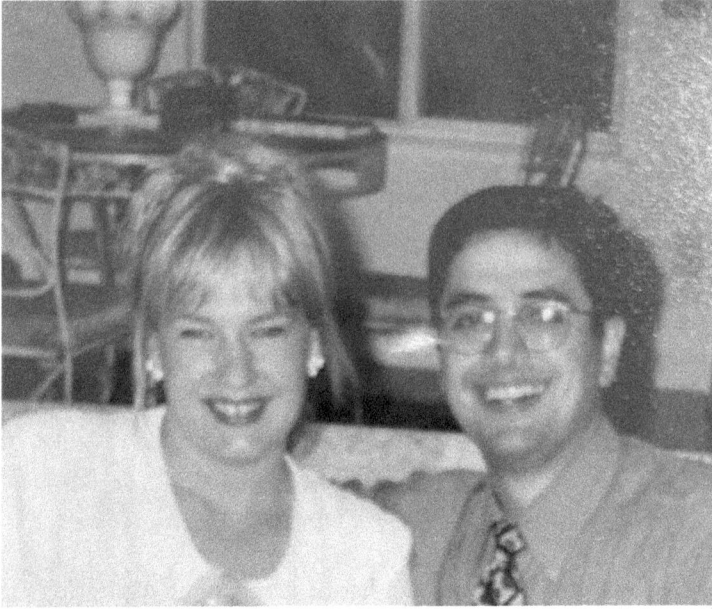

My new husband—Kris, pictured above—headed off early each morning to work as a retail pharmacist as I navigated the foreign skills of cooking meals and running a house. But even more difficult was figuring out my life's direction. The local community hospital did not hire me to join their team, even after a compelling presentation on how my Stanford-gained skills could improve diabetes care at their facility. I felt bereft. I was lonely and jobless, contemplating resuming my role as a floor nurse. Then, a brochure arrived in the mail that changed everything.

Do you believe the universe sends you messages, notes, or signs to help guide your way? I am a big believer in signs from the universe, and I really needed one. As I was losing my sense of direction and leaning into self-doubt, the message I needed was delivered to my doorstep.

Academy Medical Training Company was hiring healthcare professionals to speak on various topics. They needed specialty speakers to teach at healthcare conferences nationwide, where attendees could gain knowledge and earn continuing education credit. Speakers were required to teach for eight hours during the day, fly to another state that night, and wake up early to teach eight hours again the next day. Earning our $5000 weekly stipend required doing this for five days straight on little sleep and lousy food. I traveled light and only packed a carry-on with my speaking outfits, my handout, and a slide carousel. We went "on tour" once a month and then rested for three weeks.

As exhausting as this experience was, it allowed me to practice different approaches to teaching healthcare professionals from various walks of life across the country. I learned valuable lessons from the attendees' questions, comments, and facial expressions. I kept adjusting my slides and content until I was a well-tuned training machine. I taught through sleep deprivation, in dingy conference rooms, during storms, when the microphone wasn't working, and when I thought I couldn't stand one more minute. But I gave it my all no matter what, just like I had back in Ying's Kitchen.

Between Academy Medical and other speaking engagements, I had clocked over 1000 hours of public speaking by the end of that year. I was well on my way to mastery, which, according to Malcolm Gladwell's book *Outliers*, requires spending 10,000 hours on your craft. The notion is that consistent practice over time leads to mastery. Even if you don't reach that exact number of hours, deliberate practice, feedback, and improvement will help you fine-tune your craft and build confidence. Over the course of that year, my self-confidence grew, and I began to thrive on speaking and sharing my message of compassionate diabetes care.

Out of Your Comfort Zone and Into Your Future

Before I knew it, this demanding speaking experience forced me out of my comfort zone and launched me into my future. In addition to mastering public speaking, I learned to wrestle with difficult feedback from course evaluations. Imagine looking at hundreds of post-course evaluations after pouring your heart into your teaching and then sitting with reflections on your course, most affirming, but some going right to the heart. Determining which criticism is genuine and helpful and which is nothing more than petty comments from a frustrated individual takes time to fine-tune. This is true in life, too. When you ask for feedback, you are moved to take an honest look at yourself to recognize and address areas ready for growth and reflection.

Have you read feedback after a lecture or performance and only noticed the criticisms, amplifying the negative personal comments in your head and downplaying the mostly fantastic feedback? The negative comments would get lodged in my chest, encouraging the monster of self-doubt to get big and loud. However, with time, I learned to release the mean statements and adjust my content and teaching style based on the constructive feedback I received.

Presenting live also revealed something magical: I love public speaking! The meaningful connections I made with the audience through my words and intentions felt healing—for both me and the attendees. I discovered that speaking about diabetes care and translating complicated scientific concepts into understandable human terms gave me deep satisfaction. In addition, it provided me with a microphone to address the judgment and shame often attached to diabetes care, and I wanted to find a way to do it more.

If an opportunity comes your way and you are looking at the pros and cons, lean toward YES. Moving toward action and taking the risk usually outweighs the benefits of sticking with the status quo. By saying YES to traversing the country and teaching classes in different time zones in small conference rooms that smelled of smoke, I earned a hard-won epiphany: I could create my own version of a diabetes education training company and take back the reins of my life.

In 1998, I met with my husband and best friends and pitched the idea of launching a company. With their enthusiastic support, we sketched out a business plan, laying the foundation for my future. "Diabetes Education Services" was born on a wine-soaked napkin with my most trusted life advisors. That moment launched me into the next phase of my life.

In this chapter, I am cheering you on to take that risk and open the door to your possibilities. It's time to tackle that new initiative, design an innovative program, or make that proposal to your boss. Of course, this whole notion of finally doing that "thing" you have been dreaming about could be terrifying, exhilarating, or a little bit of both. But remember, on the other side of fear lies an incredible sense of empowerment and sheer badassery. There are so many reasons not to leap into a new version of yourself, like past trauma, self-doubt, impostor syndrome, lack of resources, shyness, and fear of failure. These reasons are real and valid; they are a part of you. But they don't define you. You can't make these reasons disappear, but you can stand next to them and let them know that they will not stop you.

Kickstart Your Dream Project

Let's say you are finally ready to kick off that dream project you have been thinking about for a few months or years. You feel stuck because considering the first steps of this project causes an unexpected combination of dread and excitement. Yet, you notice you daydream about it in those quiet moments and find yourself making lists of what needs to happen next to get it started. That is a sign that you are ready for the next step: committing this idea to paper and carefully evaluating the pros, cons, and feasibility of this dream. This idea doesn't have to be grandiose and life-changing; it simply needs your complete commitment and a ton of desire to make it come to life. And, just a warning, this little baby will probably take more time and effort than you initially imagined. That is okay! Think of all the lessons you GET to learn along the way.

You have it within you to take the wheel, press on the gas, and drive this car down the less-traveled road. No matter what type of facility you work in, you will notice things that need fixing, improvement, revitalization, or recreation. This is your chance to say YES, to take that leap of faith, get uncomfortable, put your best self forward, press the pedal, and go for it!

How do you feel about this idea? Excited? Scared? Apprehensive? All of those are perfectly valid and normal. Feeling fearful when thinking about taking action can signify that you are deeply invested in something meaningful. Take a moment to reconnect with your project's purpose, like improving patient care, increasing access to services, or expanding your knowledge. This can help ground you so you can refocus on why this project matters. You are engaging in courage by identifying something that is missing or broken and taking the risk of saying "out loud" that it needs fixing. This act of bravery can improve care and be a source of healing for you, your colleagues, and the people you serve.

What crazy dream have you locked away because it seemed too outlandish to yourself or others? Now's the time to pull it back out of the safety box and reconsider its potential. Let's say you pursue this idea, and it doesn't exactly work out as you hoped. What's the worst that will happen? You could end up birthing a different version of this dream. Or you could learn something important about yourself that has been hidden all this time. By daring to believe in the possibility and taking steps toward your dream, you'll gain insights about who you are—insights that may prove just as valuable, if not more so, than achieving the dream itself.

Tune Into Your Body Wisdom When Facing Big Decisions

The next piece of advice may cause you to question my sanity, wisdom, and business acumen. So, before I share this most critical recommendation with you (besides the absolute necessity of creating a detailed plan), I want to reassure you that using this secret sauce strategy in my own company has always steered me in the right direction. This approach is the north star that keeps me TRUE to my vision without settling for less. It has informed me if I am veering off track or compromising my values and mission. I ask you one small favor: take this action before you move forward on your dream project and this madcap adventure that is lodged in your brain.

Write your vision clearly, including your mission statement and overall goals. Include the steps needed to actualize your plan and what and who you will need to enlist to make this dream come to life. Write down the benefits and the drawbacks. Take a close look at the finances to ensure your idea is fiscally feasible.

Now, visualize your idea in detail and imagine it entirely in your mind's eye. Do a deep dive into your body and ask it carefully to consider if this zany adventure feels right. Keep breathing and monitor your body responses from toe to head.

What is your body telling you? Does it feel tense and uncomfortable, with sweaty palms and gastrointestinal distress? Are your feet tight with an overall sense of "this doesn't feel good?" If your body feels out of harmony simply thinking about your idea, then this plan for your future is probably not the best fit. Ask yourself what changes are needed to make it align with your values or to create a sense of harmony in your body. Then, rewrite your plan, imagine it coming to fruition, and see how it feels in your body.

You may have the opposite experience. When you envision your plan, even with the pros and cons, does your body feel relaxed and energized, excited by the prospect of this idea, and ready to get started? If yes, this is a strong sign you are moving in the right direction! Trust this feeling and keep checking in with yourself as you take steps to move your dream forward. Along those lines, give yourself permission to sit with ideas and let them percolate. You may even want to share them with people you trust to take them for a test drive. Keep listening to your body's response and trust yourself.

For the past thirty years, when making important decisions, I have been tuning into my mind-body wisdom with great success. Tuning into your body and emotions to assess whether a plan aligns with your values and long-term goals keeps you on track. By balancing practical considerations with this internal check-in, you move toward choices that make sense logically and feel right on a deeper level. This approach echoes the shared and ancient sentiment, "Trust Your Gut," but it is more significant than that. This saying could be read more fully: "Trust your mind-body wisdom." I learned to trust this approach more and more over time, and other research has verified these findings.

As part of her Wayfinder Life Coach Training, the esteemed Dr. Martha Beck teaches how to access this wisdom by using your body as a "compass" to find your way to a life you love. Dr. Beck states, "Our bodies patiently persist in telling us the truth, and learning to listen to this inner knowing helps us make sound choices in any situation."

This approach has given me the courage to figure out my worth when asking for a speaking fee, helped me determine if I should propose a new project idea, and absolutely encouraged me to kick off my DiabetesEd Online University. This last action launched my online university that propelled my company into the next level of success over 15 years ago.

Examples of Bringing the Dream to Life

Perhaps you want to start a program that combines diabetes and dancing. Or maybe you have the harebrained idea to organize a Diabetes Walk to create a scholarship fund or start your own side hustle or business. Let's look at some examples of how these seeds of ideas can become your reality.

Example 1: Building a Scholarship Program

At a rural northern California hospital, our team created a thriving and popular Diabetes Self-Management Program recognized by the

American Diabetes Association. This four-session program included education on self-management by a team of RNs and RDs, plus dancing, group sharing, healthy snacks, and a bag of diabetes swag for program graduates. However, we faced a serious barrier. Many folks with diabetes in our community couldn't participate because they did not have adequate insurance coverage to attend. Because of Medicare rules, we had to charge everyone the same price, which would be cost-prohibitive for those paying cash.

Our diabetes education team was ready to break down this barrier and ensure everyone who wanted diabetes self-care information could receive it.

We met with the accounting department, which suggested creating a Diabetes Scholarship Fund that could be used to pay the diabetes class fee for those without insurance. Creating the fund was easy enough, but we needed money to add to it. We asked colleagues and our diabetes participants if they had ideas about how to raise funds for this scholarship program. Someone came up with the idea of holding a walk for diabetes in our community. We gathered community leaders to work out the logistics and marketing.

Within a year, we had our "Strides for Diabetes Walk," which raised more than enough money to fill our scholarship fund coffers. This popular event was more than a walk; it was a community event we held annually for over a decade. People arrived in teams with strollers, wheelchairs, and costumes, all excited to contribute and raise awareness. We had our very own DJ, music, healthy snacks, and dancing, plus we raised enough money to ensure we never turned anyone away from our diabetes self-management program.

In the picture on the next page, our Feather River Hospital Strides for Diabetes Team is dressed up in a country theme as part of our team costume. Our annual tradition was to take a quick photo under the balloon arch before all the walkers arrived.

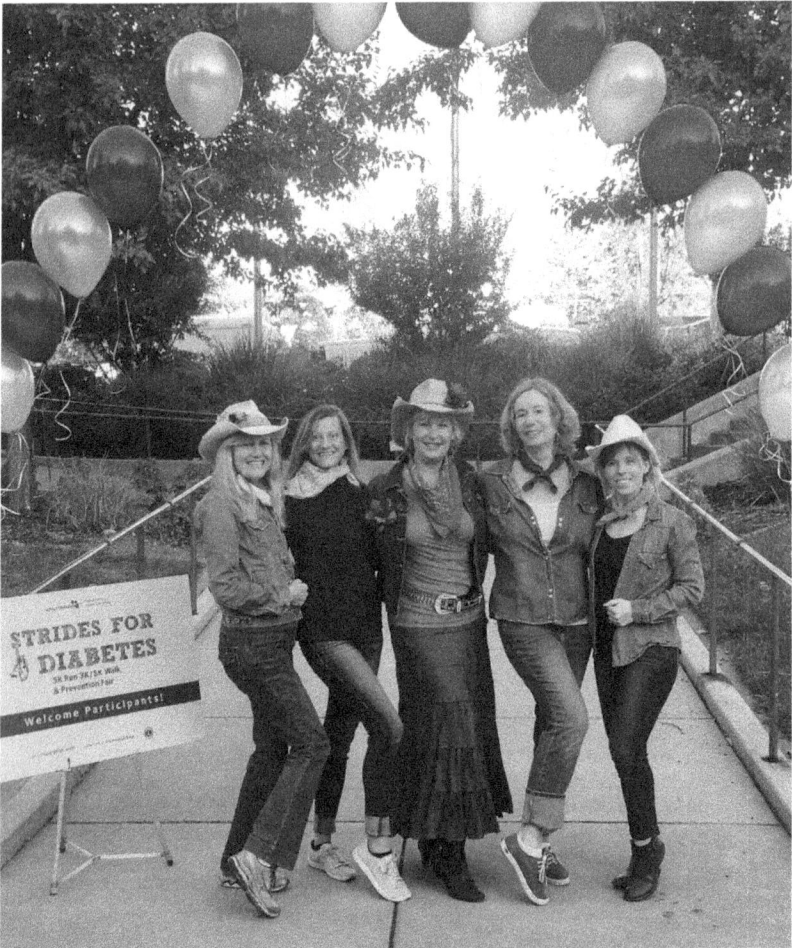

From left to right, Dawn DeSoto, Lisa Martens, Beverly Thomassian, Caroline Kelly, and Jenae Hawkins.

As a team dedicated to providing care, our vision was to ensure everyone could attend our classes. By seeking input, working out the details, and making sure it all felt right, we moved forward and raised funds while bringing a community together. This is just one example of a dream that came to life out of necessity, led by a small team of dedicated diabetes enthusiasts. I encourage you to think big and not let barriers hinder providing the best care for people with diabetes.

When I reflect on what we accomplished, Margaret Mead's quote says it best: "Never doubt that a small group of thoughtful, committed individuals can change the world. In fact, it's the only thing that ever has."

Example 2: Dancing Out Diabetes

One morning, while listening to dance jams on an iPod shuffle she had won at an AADE conference, Theresa Garnero, a diabetes specialist who had been recognized as Diabetes Educator of the Year, felt the tug between her love for dancing and her dedication to diabetes education. As she hesitated to pull the earbuds out and head to work, an idea struck her—why not combine her two passions? That moment became the genesis of Dance Out Diabetes, a groundbreaking, nonprofit initiative that brought the clinic to the dance floor.

The concept was simple yet innovative: create a space where people with all types of diabetes, along with their family and friends, could come together to dance, have fun, and access resources for managing and preventing diabetes. The program included health screenings like A1C, BP, and other metrics, and diabetes educators supported participants in a joyous, nonjudgmental environment. The monthly intervention was held at a local community center. It featured a DJ and numerous boxes of medical equipment—carefully stored to ensure the integrity of testing supplies—unloaded from a packed car and schlepped to the educator tables by an incredible team of volunteers. Dance styles varied with each session, ranging from hip-hop to salsa, Bollywood, and even Michael Jackson's "Thriller," with expert instructors leading the group every month.

Dance Out Diabetes was intentionally inclusive, welcoming participants of all ages, abilities, and diabetes types, along with their support systems. One memorable dance featured a newborn on a mat alongside a mother managing gestational diabetes, individuals with type 1 and type 2 diabetes—including a 97-year-old—and others dedicated to diabetes prevention. Remarkably, for those with prediabetes, the health outcomes surpassed those of the Diabetes Prevention Program (DPP). Nearly all returning participants showed improvements in both health and mental well-being. Most importantly, the program brought immense joy to everyone who attended.

Over five years, the program survived on private donations, in-kind support, and an extraordinary team of volunteers. Though the program was impactful, the lack of sustained funding made it difficult to continue. In 2015, Dance Out Diabetes held its final event—a celebratory Sicilian Tarantella. Despite its closure, the program left a lasting legacy. Many participants have stayed in touch, sharing how much the experience meant to them. For Theresa, Dance Out Diabetes was a career highlight—a realized dream that seamlessly blended movement, community, and diabetes prevention and care in an unforgettable way. While the program's outcomes were published and celebrated, the smiles of participants, educators, instructors, and volunteers truly captured its impact.

Example 3: Starting Diabetes Education Services

I founded Diabetes Education Services in May 1998, just as the World Wide Web was emerging, and this new thing called "email" became a way to communicate. Initially, my one-person company focused solely on offering live courses at hospitals and conference venues nationwide. My "office" was a 10×12-foot room in our home, where I balanced writing a monthly newsletter, articles, and book chapters, updating presentation slides, and raising two energetic toddlers.

Building something of this magnitude was never a solo journey. I was fortunate to have the unwavering support of my husband and life partner, Kristapor Thomassian, and my closest friends and board members, Jane Steinberg and Jony Weiss. This incredible trio became my anchor, my sounding board, and my source of guidance as the company navigated decades of growth and change.

Through the whirlwind of those early years, their steadfast support kept me grounded in my company's mission: to empower healthcare professionals to achieve their goal of becoming certified diabetes specialists so they can deliver compassionate, person-centered care to people living with diabetes.

For the first decade, I slowly established myself as a leader in the field by hustling to speak at as many in-person training and keynote presentations as possible. With the onset of a global recession, people couldn't afford to travel to trainings, and speaking opportunities dwindled. My husband earned enough to meet our basic needs, but I wanted to contribute more. I also wanted to reach my potential and get my message out to a broader audience. My kids had entered school, so I had more free time to grow my company and was ready to take on a new challenge. I mailed thousands of brochures to encourage healthcare professionals to sign up for our live courses or hire me as a speaker. Below is a snippet of one of my early headshots on a flyer from 1999 that marketed our company's services and products.

PRESIDENT, DES

Author, nurse, educator and clinician, Beverly Dyck Thomassian has specialized in diabetes management for the past 10 years. She has been awarded Board Certification in Advanced Diabetes Management and has been published in the American Journal of Nursing, NurseWeek, Progress for Cardiovascular Nursing, Stanford Nurse and Japanese Journal of Nursing.

Over time, I started growing a list of mailing and, eventually, email addresses, which made connecting with our community much easier. In 2010, I made the terrifying decision to create the DiabetesEd Online University learning platform so students could take CE training courses online. This doesn't sound revolutionary today, but it bordered on madness at the time. I only had one part-time employee who helped with product shipping and answering phone calls, and I was a diabetes content expert with limited technical knowledge. My rinky-dink website was chaotic and clunky, but I was determined to be an early adopter and a thought leader in the field.

After mulling over the idea of starting an online university and brainstorming with my three-person team, I realized that to succeed, I needed help! With tears in my eyes, I hired the wonderful Lainey Koski, a woman who had built a computer from scratch and helped launch an online start-up CE company. To get my website from chaos to harmony, I contracted with Farrell Design, a female-owned web design company that took the time to listen to and understand my company and vision. These knowledgeable, incredible women revamped my website and opened my company up to the wider diabetes community. Within months, Diabetes Education Services was discovered, and we were off and running.

Today, more than 26 years after the inception of this company, I have mentored thousands of healthcare professionals to become certified diabetes specialists. At the core of all our education and training is providing person-centered care infused with compassion and kindness. I feel proud that I have also mentored many staff members, and they have moved on to advance their careers and use their skills in new ways. Both of my boys were paid members of the Diabetes Education Team, learning from a young age about how to run a business and treat people with respect. They witnessed their mom focused and fierce, pushing through hard times and profitable times.

I have learned to write a business plan, review a profit and loss statement, and make adjustments to get back on track. I've been fortunate enough to earn enough to create a beautiful office, support my kids through college, and invest in causes I deeply believe in. Most importantly, I get to do what I love while growing the next generation of compassionate and empathetic diabetes care and education specialists.

As I give back and share the hard-earned lessons from my journey, I'm not just offering support to healthcare professionals and those I serve, I'm also receiving something profound in return. The connections formed along the way have become a powerful and essential part of my own healing.

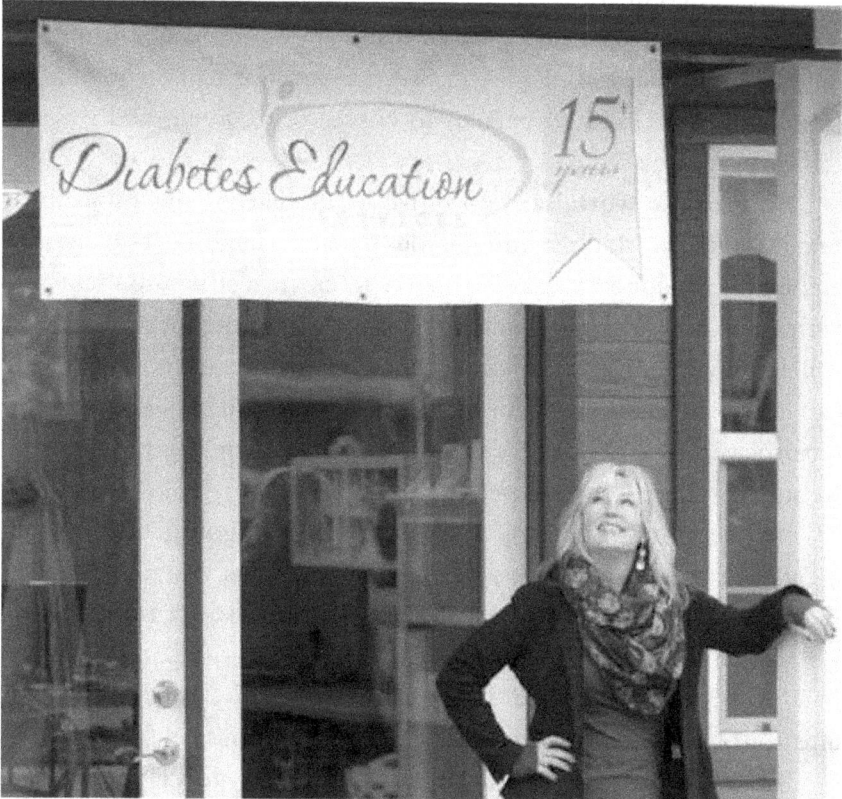

In 2013, we celebrated our 15th year by building a new office!

6 Essential Steps to Launch Your Dream Project

Your dream is different from mine, but you can learn from my mistakes to turn it into a reality. Here are six things I wish I had known when I started turning my crazy idea into a tangible business. **Have a clear and persistent vision of your goals, and ensure your program aligns with your values**. Take a retreat with yourself (or with friends you trust) and carefully ponder what is most important to you as you think through this project or program. What do you want to realize in five years, 10 years, and beyond? This is more than setting financial goals. Your answers will reveal your program's core meaning and value, and what you will feel proud standing next to. As an example, my company is a value-based business. Our goal is to provide compassionate and evidence-based diabetes education that promotes kindness and curiosity. Early on, we decided not to accept funding from diabetes-related companies to ensure our content and mission remained non-biased.

Be ready to work hard and give back. Starting this project will require you to work three times harder than expected. That's okay; that is the effort required to take flight. Try to create a structured schedule with a start and stop time, and don't forget to take time for recreation— it helps keep your creative juices flowing. Share your knowledge and expertise with others to help build community and create a sense of reciprocity. Write articles, volunteer as a podcast guest, provide free webinars, and say yes to opportunities to highlight your knowledge.

Be prepared to fail, get back up, and keep going. Starting this baby will require taking risks, trusting your instincts, and jumping into the unknown. Most of the time, ideas led by your wisdom, coupled with a strong business sense, will succeed, but every so often, they will fall flat. That is to be expected. Incorporate that hard-earned knowledge into your new, informed vision and resume your journey forward.

Keep physically fit, eat healthfully, and don't scrimp on sleep. A tired and underslept brain and body will struggle to rise to the challenge. Find ways to incorporate activity throughout the day and commit to getting adequate sleep to optimize your performance. For example, to keep active while working, I walk on a desk treadmill while creating slides, writing articles, and reading emails. I also dance weekly with a troupe, which primes my mental and physical health and improves neuroplasticity. Regular movement boosts neural integration and helps you synthesize complex concepts. Plus, it is a lot of fun!

Nurture family and friend connections. Starting a big project can be emotionally demanding. Carving out time for family and friends helps keep you grounded and provides a sense of security and belonging. They help with problem-solving and are happy to cheer you on.

Believe in yourself. When starting a new endeavor, the voice of doubt can rear its ugly head. Learn how to be your own best self-coach to remind yourself why this is important and that you have a clear vision of where you are going. Stumbles are expected and natural. Take a break, walk outside, breathe, and regroup. You got this!

Even though I have been running my company for 25 plus years, I still experience moments of doubt when building my dream. Doubt is a powerful messenger that makes me dig deeper to ensure my decision is based on sound reasoning. Sometimes, doubt is a sign that I need to practice my talk one more time before stepping onto the stage. But mostly, doubt is a piece of baggage that I can release, knowing that I have earned this moment and that I have what I need within me to make my dreams come true. I give myself permission to stand firm in my success and acknowledge that I am enough.

I Believe in Your Success

You deserve to bring your dream to life, no matter how big or small the vision. Start by clearly imagining and defining your dream. Then, get support, set realistic goals, and keep moving toward the end goal one step at a time. Take consistent action toward your dream as you listen to your body's wisdom, embrace challenges, and remain willing to adapt and learn on the journey. Make sure to reward yourself along the way and celebrate milestones. As Eleanor Roosevelt once wisely said, "The future belongs to those who believe in the beauty of their dreams."

• • •

My next chapter delves into the power of how your words and body language can either uplift or discourage the very people you are committed to serving. Imagine a healthcare setting where individuals of all backgrounds and lived experiences feel truly safe, heard, and seen—without judgment—a place where their achievements are celebrated and person-centered problem-solving is the norm. I believe in the power of this approach, and the next chapter provides plenty of examples of how to promote judgment-free care.

CHAPTER 5

The ABCs of Creating a Judgment-Free Connection

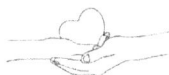

*"Out beyond ideas of wrongdoing and right doing,
there is a field. I'll meet you there."*

—Rumi

My first patient at the clinic that morning was Maria, a young woman with diabetes who had started wearing a continuous glucose monitor for the past week. This sensor was meant to ease the burden of pricking her fingers three to four times daily to measure her blood glucose before injecting insulin. After a quick hug and hello, I asked Maria how she was doing. She held her glucose reader away from her and faced it toward me with her head down. She said with tears, "I can't stand to look at the numbers."

When I asked her why, she blurted out, "Because I am failing. My numbers always go up after I eat."

I touched her knee, took a deep breath, and reassured her.

"You are not failing. Everyone's blood glucose levels go up after eating."

She wiped her tears and looked me in the eye. "Really?"

"Yes, really," I said gently. "That's a completely expected result after eating." I continued, "You are not failing. Your pancreas isn't working right." A simple but powerful reframe: blame the pancreas, not the person.

That brief exchange became a moment of transformation. Maria had been carrying around silent shame and self-judgment, and with a few carefully chosen words, her perspective began to shift. She realized she wasn't failing . . . and she wasn't alone.

How many times have you met people with diabetes who are disheartened, discouraged, and judging themselves for their weight, their blood glucose levels, what they eat or don't eat, and a million other things? They may hesitate to express their feelings of failure, worried they're "letting you down."

One of your most important roles as a healthcare professional is creating a safe space where people can share their stories without judgment.

Like Maria, many people living with diabetes experience distress when their glucose levels aren't in the target range. However, diabetes is a condition no one chooses, and it demands constant attention with no days off. Managing diabetes is complex, with outcomes shaped by far more than motivation or discipline alone.

Sadly, some people walk away from healthcare visits feeling even worse, especially when healthcare professionals (HCPs) reinforce negative self-talk by focusing too heavily on shortcomings. This approach can cause disconnection from the HCP relationship and decrease participation in healthcare.

This chapter explores how the way you speak, listen, and respond can profoundly shape the care experience. Every interaction holds the potential to either build trust and safety or, unintentionally, create distance and reinforce feelings of shame. You'll discover practical strategies to move away from judgment and stigma and reinvigorate your practice through a compassionate, person-centered approach. By implementing this simple ABC approach, you can transform routine encounters into opportunities for healing and connection, both for the people you care for and yourself.

You Can Help Move Away from Shame and Stigma

Of all the chronic conditions I have worked with, diabetes carries a disproportionate load of stigma and shaming by well-meaning HCPs who often feel compelled to point out where the person with diabetes is falling short instead of recognizing all the actions they are already taking.

John arrived at the clinic excited that his time in range using a sensor had been above 60% for the past month. But when his HCP looked at the ambulatory glucose report, they shook their head and said, "Well, you know your time in range should be at least 70%? Keep trying to cut back on your carbs and come back in three months."

The HCP likely felt they were conveying factual information about the standards of care and motivating John to do "better." But to John, who was already trying his best to manage diabetes, these comments from a trusted healthcare professional led to feeling ashamed, judged, and embarrassed as he concluded that he was failing at managing diabetes.

What is the long-term consequence of this brief HCP-patient interaction and thousands of other interactions like it? Chances are, John will likely feel discouraged and distressed about diabetes and continue to feel like he is a failure. He may be reluctant to make his next appointment or lose interest in trying to lower his glucose levels. He might start to feel hopeless about ever being able to manage his diabetes effectively. By focusing on numbers and "facts" instead of the thoughts and feelings of the person standing in front of them, the HCP may have unwittingly discouraged John from continuing to receive care and engaging with diabetes, leading to worse health outcomes down the road.

With misinformed intentions, the HCP may feel that judgment and shame will serve as a motivator to move people with diabetes forward. Unfortunately, research shows shame and scare tactics close the door to follow-up and return visits. Instead of motivating those with diabetes, these tactics can increase feelings of hopelessness and low self-esteem, intensify diabetes distress, and increase no-show rates.

A recent survey of over 2,600 people with diabetes across eight countries revealed that nearly 40% of missed doctor's appointments are due to stigma or shame. Brene Brown describes shame as a "painful feeling of believing you are flawed and unworthy, often leading to self-criticism and a sense of inadequacy or unworthiness."

Many healthcare professionals incorrectly assume that people with diabetes are not reaching their goals due to a lack of effort. If they "just tried hard enough," they could reach the recommended time-in-range target. Unfortunately, this false belief can build a wall of misunderstanding between the HCP and the person with diabetes.

In this example, John was hoping for the simple recognition that he was achieving time in range most of the time. Let's replay this interaction using a person-centered approach.

How You Can Incorporate a Person-Centered Approach

John arrived at the clinic excited that his time in range using a sensor was above 60% for the past month. When his HCP looked at the ambulatory glucose report, they smiled, looked at John, and said, "Wow, John, I can see you are making an effort to improve your blood glucose levels. What have you been doing differently to get your time in range above sixty percent?"

How easy was that? Look at all the positive things that happened in that 30-second reflection by the HCP using a person-centered approach. First, John's work was recognized by his HCP, whom he looks up to. The HCP uses body language (smiling and looking John in the eyes) and acknowledging words, "you are making an effort to improve glucose levels," to affirm John's effort. The HCP then shifts to curiosity and asks John to share his expertise in his health. "What have you been doing to improve your time in range?" John is thrilled to answer this question and shares that he has been bike riding after dinner to improve his post-dinner glucose. Plus, he has been taking his medication every day and trying to drink more water.

The HCP then states, "It seems like you have identified several things that lower your blood glucose. Great effort. What would you like to work on for your next visit?"

John shares that he plans to continue the changes he has already made and start packing his lunch to see if that decreases his after-meal glucose elevations. John leaves the visit feeling heard, seen, and hopeful. He is excited to keep working on his diabetes self-management.

By recognizing John's expertise in his own health, values, and preferences, and by acknowledging the progress and effort he has already made, the HCP has sent a clear message that they believe in John's ability to manage his diabetes. The HCP refrained from judgment and instead focused on John's strengths, effort, and goals. By engaging in curiosity, they elicited actions John was already taking and explored what he would like to address in the future.

This approach is beneficial not only for the person receiving care but also for the HCP. Instead of dreaming up what you think will help the person, you can tap into their expertise and self-knowledge. A person-centered approach also leads to less HCP burnout since you connect with people authentically, releasing yourself from being responsible for their choices.

Forging genuine connections can be done with a simple **ABC** approach. **A**ssess and **A**cknowledge something the person is succeeding at and **A**sk with curiosity how they accomplished this behavior change. Identify any **B**arriers that may be blocking their forward movement. Then, determine what **C**hange they would like to work on with **C**ompassion and **C**uriosity.

In the end, a person-centered approach doesn't only support the person with diabetes. It also supports the healthcare professional by fostering authentic connection, shared responsibility, and a greater sense of purpose in your work.

Addressing Distress and Emotions - Reignite Your Fire

The ABC framework is a good starting point, but it is missing the **D** for Diabetes Distress and **E** for Emotions. As we continue this discussion, let's add those two concepts.

I was invited to participate in the EMBARK (Behavioral Approaches to Reducing Diabetes Distress and Improving HbA1c) study as a diabetes specialist. My job was to provide diabetes self-management coaching to people living with type 1 diabetes based on the research protocol. The lead researchers and diabetes psychologists, Dr. Larry Fisher and Dr. Susan Guzman, focused on addressing common emotional responses to living with diabetes, including distress.

The findings of the EMBARK trial confirmed that prioritizing emotions to support individuals living with diabetes resulted in significant reductions in diabetes distress AND A1C levels.

As a healthcare professional, you may tend to focus on problem-solving around lifestyle and medications, thinking that if you get those right, diabetes distress will improve along with glucose levels. However, the study results show that it is time to flip that idea on its head. By addressing emotional distress, people are better able to deal with the demands of diabetes self-management and improve their A1C levels.

Diabetes distress acts as a brake that stops people from taking steps to improve their health. By addressing difficult emotions, like fear of hypoglycemia, complications, or feelings of failure, the brake can be released, and the person can move forward. Let's reprioritize our checklist of diabetes topics and move into the heart of providing effective diabetes care by assessing and addressing distress early on. You can access free Diabetes Distress Scales on this website: https://www.diabetesdistress.org.

If you don't have the Diabetes Distress Scale, a quick strategy to check in with people's emotions is to ask them one of these questions:

- "What is the most difficult part of living with diabetes for you?"

- "What are your greatest concerns about your diabetes?"
- "How is your diabetes getting in the way of other things in your life right now?"

The year I spent coaching participants in the EMBARK trial re-energized me about the power of providing person-centered care. It reinforced the importance of prioritizing emotional well-being as a core part of effective diabetes support. This experience reminded me that the job of healthcare professionals is not to provide all the answers. We need to help people with diabetes discover the solution to their problems and instill in them the self-confidence that they are the ones best equipped to find the answer in the future.

The EMBARK program proved so effective that the research team felt passionate about sharing these approaches with our healthcare colleagues. We developed a training initiative called Revive 5. I'm honored to co-teach this program alongside two of my mentors and pioneers in the field of diabetes distress—Susan Guzman, PhD, and Larry Fisher, PhD. Their depth of knowledge and humanistic approach to empowering individuals with diabetes is truly extraordinary.

Creating Judgment-Free Zones

Feelings of blame and judgment in healthcare are common. They are almost like unconscious thought patterns built into our medical model. However, when judgment takes the lead, it can prevent trust from forming and healing from taking root.

By becoming aware of your inner dialogue and exchanging judgment with curiosity, you actively engage in a more mindful practice and start meeting people where they are, with compassion. Curiosity leans in with openness, seeking to understand rather than to label. It invites connection, discovery, and the possibility of seeing things, especially people, in a new light.

Seeing people through the lens of curiosity brings out the best in you, matching the reason you entered healthcare in the first place—to help with healing. The goal is to give yourself permission to set those feelings of judgment aside and see the person as they are in that moment—complex, capable, and worthy. When you approach others with genuine curiosity instead of criticism, you create space for healing to unfold for them and yourself.

Below are examples of comments from well-meaning HCPs and suggested reframes to promote a more person-centered, curiosity-based response. Please feel free to steal and share these responses as needed.

HCP: "Have you seen how much fruit JR is eating? Don't they know they have diabetes?"

Your evidence-based reframe: "People with diabetes are encouraged to enjoy these nutrient-dense, high-fiber foods daily. Fruits are a healthier choice than processed treats, and the American Diabetes Association (ADA) Standards recommend people with diabetes eat three servings a day."

HCP: "No wonder their glucose is so high. This patient is non-compliant; they only take their insulin four times a week instead of every day."

Your curiosity-based reframe: "This person is managing to take their insulin four times a week. Let's see if we can figure out why it's working on those days but not on the other three days. We might need to adjust the plan to match their life."

HCP: "Of course they have diabetes; look at how much they weigh."

Your evidence-based reframe: "There are a lot of individuals who have extra weight and never get diabetes. The expression of type 2 diabetes is due to a complex interplay between genetics, environment, social determinants of health, trauma, and age. Diabetes incidence and prevalence are a reflection of the overall health of the community and the lived experiences of the individual. A higher rate of diabetes in a given region is an indicator of health inequity and is often coupled with systemic racism. Reducing the rates of diabetes needs to start with healing our communities and building bridges between healthcare professionals and the people we serve."

When you provide non-judgmental care infused with curiosity and compassion, you honor the strengths of the people you serve. You also infuse your consciousness with kindness in place of judgment. This approach leads to more effective care and healing that flows both ways. As you provide healing care to others, you also send your psyche a message of compassion and reassurance that you will be okay.

Create a Judgement Free Zone – Roll out the Carpet of Acceptance

There are no bad or good blood glucose numbers.
There is no such thing as cheating.
You are not failing at your diabetes.
It is not your fault you have diabetes.
Thank you for showing up today.

The New Language of Diabetes – Uplifting People with Diabetes

Language packages our shared experiences into symbols shared and digested by the presenter and listener. In 2017, a consensus report formalized the importance of language in daily practice. The paper, "The

Use of Language in Diabetes Care and Education," emphasizes the critical role words play in diabetes management and engagement. The paper advocates for adopting respectful, nonjudgmental, and empowering language to foster positive person-centered relationships. The report outlines recommendations that address the need for reduced stigma and improved communication in diabetes care.

Based on the language guidelines, here is a short list of words and phrases you can ditch from your vocabulary. First, the term "diabetic" is officially off-limits. A person with diabetes is not defined by their disease. They are a person living with a chronic condition or a person with diabetes. Next, say goodbye to the phrases "non-compliant" or "non-adherent." Instead, focus on what people are accomplishing. "JR is taking their medications on weekdays." Retire the word "test" blood glucose and replace it with the term "check." After all, blood glucose levels do not receive a pass or fail grade. They simply provide information on the current glucose levels in the person's body.

As educators, advocates, spouses, friends, and HCPs, our use of language can profoundly affect the self-views of people living with diabetes every day. We can help change the current paradigm by using language that lifts people up instead of communications that can lead them to feel defeated.

In addition to body language and active listening, you can reassure people that diabetes isn't about doing everything right; it's about creating realistic expectations, considering each person's situation. You can encourage people with diabetes to release the goal of perfection and strive for "healthy good enough," a phrase used by a thought leader and colleague, Susan Guzman, PhD. The language you choose when coaching people with diabetes is powerful and can have a lasting impact on perceptions and behavior.

This final section offers a practical summary you can apply in your clinical practice to deliver compassionate and effective diabetes care while leaving you with a sense of fulfillment at the end of the day.

The ABCs of Judgment-Free Person-Centered Care
A: Ask, Assess, Acknowledge

During that first sit-down meeting, listen carefully to the individual's story to find out how they feel about their diabetes and what they want to focus on. Engaging in active listening is considered a therapeutic intervention on its own. Active listening includes asking questions, rephrasing to ensure you got it right, providing encouragement, and being curious about the person's feelings and health issues. This is also the perfect time to explore Diabetes Distress and Emotions. People often tear up when they share their stories; that is okay. I always have a box of tissues in my office, just in case. Be reassured that you don't have to fix anything; your job is to listen, acknowledge, and remind folks that they are not alone. You want the person to know that you see and hear them.

For the following few examples, I will use an outdated phrase. See if you can conjure up a more person-centered approach.

Outdated phrase: "Your A1C is really high."

Person-centered approach: "I see that your A1C is 9.3%. I am curious, what is your A1C goal?"

Here, you want to use neutral words and physiology instead of words that can invoke feelings of shame. Avoid using the phrase "really high" if possible and say "above target" instead. This more neutral approach can help steer away from feelings of failure since many individuals base their success on glucose results. In truth, it is impossible to achieve perfect blood glucose levels with a disease where the pancreas has lost over half of its insulin-producing beta cells. Since the human body is dynamic, despite an individual's best efforts, blood glucose levels can go above or below target at any given moment. Perfection is not required! The goal is to balance quality of life and diabetes management or achieve a status of "healthy good enough."

Outdated phrase: "You can control your diabetes by exercising and eating right."

Person-centered approach: "Keeping active can help you manage your blood glucose levels. Is there an activity you enjoy doing?"

HCPs often dole out instructions to get moving and eat healthfully. You have heard these recommendations a million times from health experts. But what does this mean for the individual sitting across from you? First, you can start by briefly summarizing the benefits of movement: "Taking a ten-minute walk after meals can lower your blood glucose levels." Hyping up the "why" may help people feel more motivated to give it a try.

The next part is crucial to increase success. Ask THEM if there are any activities they enjoy doing. You will see their face light up as they share activities they enjoy or remember activities they loved doing but have left by the wayside. Bingo. Now, ask them if they could bring that activity into their present life and explore what that would look like. You may even collaborate on creating an incredibly achievable goal so they can experience a win. "I will dance in my house for ten minutes on Monday, Wednesday, and Saturday."

When conducting the initial assessment, you aim to assess, ask questions, and actively listen. By limiting one-way instruction and exploring solutions that the person holds within, you can unlock strategies that are most likely to be successful and sustained.

B: Barriers

Barriers to care are often mislabeled as non-compliance or non-adherence. It's time to relinquish this outdated framework and focus on the self-management behaviors the person with diabetes *is* achieving. Focus on facts rather than judgments. Start with where the person is and support them with problem-solving by engaging your curiosity and asking questions. Below is another example.

Outdated phrase: "MJ is non-compliant and is refusing to take her metformin medication."

Person-centered approach: "MJ hasn't started taking their metformin because they heard from their friends that it can cause kidney problems."

When meeting with an individual who isn't taking their medication, the most crucial actions are exploring why they are not and considering their valid concerns. Pay careful attention to your body language and tone of voice since this may be a very sensitive topic for the individual, especially if they are struggling with financial limitations. Many times, people don't start medications due to fear of the side effects that they have read or heard about from a friend. In this situation, you need to acknowledge their fear and share information, reassuring them that the medicine is safe and encouraging them to report any side effects immediately. Other common barriers include cost, being too busy to remember to take it, not being ready to accept their diabetes, fear of low blood glucose, and many others. These reasons are legitimate and deserve an earnest conversation to acknowledge them and explore possible solutions.

When discussing medication and self-management behaviors, being curious and using non-judgmental language helps to create trust through an honest discussion. Please credit the person with diabetes for their effort and accomplishments, then ask them how they have achieved their most recent success.

Outdated phrase: "You are only testing your blood sugar three times a week?"

Person-centered approach: "It looks like you are checking your blood glucose about three times a week. Is that accurate?"

This reframing focuses on the action the person is taking instead of the action they are not taking. Many people feel that they are failing if they only check their blood glucose three times a week, but something is always better than nothing. In addition, since many of the newer diabetes medications don't cause potentially dangerous hypoglycemia, checking three times a week at different times of day, along with a quarterly A1C, may be plenty.

When meeting with people who are not reaching their goals, embark on a process of discovery by looking for barriers and identifying areas of diabetes distress. Discuss and acknowledge the emotions swirling around their choices and diabetes self-management. Finally, if they are ready, ask them if they could try to be present with tough feelings and thoughts and still choose to try a different approach. For example, instead of giving bolus insulin right away when they see blood glucose levels going above 180 after eating, could they try deep breathing or walking for 15 minutes to see if blood glucose levels stabilize?

C: Compassion and Curiosity

Have you ever met someone taking a short or extended "diabetes break" vacation? Maybe they have stopped checking their blood glucose or aren't following any meal plan. Sometimes, their diabetes distress becomes so intense that they may stop taking their medications and relinquish many aspects of their diabetes self-management. Diabetes can be exhausting to manage day in and day out, and sometimes, people need to take a break, or what I call a "diabetes vacation." Instead of judging clients who have fallen behind, lean into compassion and offer them a helping hand to get back up and keep going.

As Nelson Mandela says, "The greatest glory in living lies not in never falling, but in rising every time we fall." When people arrive at your office or call you up after one of these "falls," they trust that you will lend them a kind and gentle hand up.

Since people with diabetes often feel judged by others, providing the gift of compassion and curiosity can open unexpected doors of insight and understanding. In my experience, people with diabetes are already hard enough on themselves. Meeting them in "the field beyond wrongdoing and right doing" can give them the courage and belief to start rewriting their journey.

Even though diabetes is a self-managed condition, as an HCP, you take on the role of coach, cheerleader, supportive problem-solver, advocate, and listener. But when the "rubber hits the road," it is the person living with diabetes every day who makes the hundreds of little decisions that move them toward or away from health.

Your job is not to provide a fix for people with diabetes but to help them discover the spark, through questions and curiosity, that motivates them to move toward health. Once the spark is discovered, only one person can ignite it. Your job is to stand close by holding the match.

People with diabetes face real-life barriers that can ignite feelings of discouragement and despair. You can help them recognize how hard they are on themselves and encourage them to explore this self-criticism. Remind them that having diabetes is not their fault and perfection is not expected. By modeling kindness, understanding, and compassion, you allow them to be gentler and more forgiving self-coaches.

Considering the Diabetes Connection as a Sacred Space

Have the stories of people living with diabetes stayed with you long after the conversation ended? Have their words, struggles, and triumphs echoed in your thoughts, quietly influencing the way you provide care? Listening to these stories isn't simply an exchange of information; it's an invitation into someone's lived experience.

When we truly listen, with presence and without judgment, we enter a sacred space within diabetes care, where healing transcends clinical roles and traditional hierarchies. In these moments, connection becomes the medicine. The person receiving care feels seen, heard, and valued. And something extraordinary happens for us as HCPs, too. We are reminded of our purpose. We feel reconnected to our humanity.

This is the heart of healing that moves both ways. A mutual exchange of trust, compassion, and insight that nourishes both the person living with diabetes and the one offering support.

I am optimistic about the future of healthcare and envision a time when people of all backgrounds and lived experiences feel safe, valued, and free from fear of judgment. In these inclusive spaces, accomplishments are celebrated, and person-centered problem-solving will be the norm. I've witnessed the transformation when healthcare professionals embrace this mindset. They become more hopeful and invigorated in their day-to-day practice. By cultivating spaces rooted in curiosity and compassion, we foster healing that radiates beyond the clinic walls, enriching patients, HCPs, and entire communities.

• • •

The next chapter focuses on creating a space for healing and self-expression. I hope you'll be delighted to discover how creative pursuits can do far more than bring joy. They can ignite new ideas, inspire unexpected solutions, and awaken an imagination that may have been quietly waiting for permission to emerge. As you read on, I hope to light a spark that encourages you to embrace your creativity without judgment or expectation, allowing it to open doors to unexpected discoveries.

CHAPTER 6

The Power of Self-Expression & Creative Endeavors

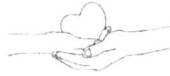

"Each of us is a creative being. Whether or not we recognize it,
we all have the potential to bring beauty,
meaning, and healing into the world."

— *Julia Cameron*

Did you know that Nobel Prize recipients are nearly three times more likely to engage in creative hobbies than their scientific counterparts?

Theoretical physicist Albert Einstein often played the violin when he encountered challenges in his theoretical work. He believed that music helped him think creatively and tap into his subconscious, enabling breakthroughs such as the theory of relativity.

Marie Curie, a two-time Nobel laureate for physics in 1903 and chemistry in 1911, went for frequent walks in the countryside, which allowed her to reflect and rejuvenate. These moments of tranquility likely helped her maintain focus during the grueling work of isolating radioactive elements.

Richard Feynman, Nobel laureate for physics in 1965, a bongo player who regularly performed in orchestra pits, solved nagging scientific problems using "acoustic images."

The statistics back up the stories. Scientists who are Nobel laureates are:

- 22 times more likely than typical scientists to perform, sing, or act in their spare time
- 12 times more likely to write fiction, plays, poetry, or short stories
- 5 times more likely to engage in crafting, woodworking, mechanics, or glassblowing
- 7 times more likely to enjoy designing, painting, drawing, or sculpting

Why are Nobel Prize winners more likely to have artistic hobbies? It's because they're simply more open to having hobbies. They are more open to novel experiences and often turn to their creative endeavors when working through challenges. These seemingly unrelated scientific pursuits and personal hobbies can open doors for scientists to cross-pollinate ideas across different fields, enabling them to gain fresh perspectives and uncover new insights.

Now, you may not be working toward securing the title of a Nobel laureate. Still, you might be interested in learning the secrets of expanding your mind, creating new connections, and better integrating the two sides of your brain hemispheres to provide better care or nurture your inner life. You may be wondering how having an artistic hobby or winning a Nobel Prize in science relates to excelling as a diabetes specialist or healthcare professional.

As a healthcare professional, you have likely lived through difficult experiences or witnessed profound suffering firsthand. Plenty of science supports the idea that engaging in creative pursuits offers an outlet to express complex emotions that are not accessible through words alone. The act of playing an instrument, taking an art class, exploring nature, or playing the bongo drums may provide a gateway to address unrequited trauma or pain, helping you to become more fully aware and present with your feelings.

This healing and self-awareness allow you to connect more fully and authentically with the people you work with and the individuals you serve. Like Einstein, Curie, and Feynman, getting out of the lab (and your head) encourages mind roaming and the opportunity to make unexpected connections that can help with problem-solving and innovation. I've lost count of how many work challenges I've resolved and moments of inspiration I've experienced while trekking through the Sierra Wilderness, building my pond, or balancing a sword on my head.

As my close friend and Professor of Public Health at USC, Jane Steinberg, PhD, beautifully describes, "I have played flute and piano since I was a small kid. In the last few years, starting at age sixty, I decided to up my game and dedicate more attention to playing flute with a focus on improvisational jazz, one of my favorite musical art forms. Jazz is a tricky beast. It is free-flowing and entirely improvisational, yet you need to know those chords, changes, and scales! While I am re-learning the theory and mechanics of jazz, I am also playing by ear and enjoying the sheer joy of making beautiful harmonic melodies (even if they come by surprise). I hope that at some point, I can fully integrate the two parts of my brain for more seamless playing. I also participate in an adult improv (acting) class once per month with friends.

"The combination of these artistic experiences has unlocked something in my brain that has noticeably impacted my workflow. Listening carefully for chord changes and focusing on musical notes has translated into a renewed ability to concentrate for more extended periods in my job without getting so easily distracted. I seem to remember dates and facts more readily, and I credit this to my musical immersion in memorizing scales, modes, and chords. I look forward to seeing where these intersecting improvisational experiences take me!"

Can you recall an "aha" moment when the solution to that perplexing problem was magically dropped at the doorstep of your mind? You may not have even been thinking about this difficulty with your conscious mind, but in the middle of singing in the shower, the answer arrived before you had time to rinse out your conditioner.

As you continue reading, I believe you'll be pleasantly surprised to discover that creative pursuits not only bring joy and unexpected solutions, but they may also reignite a dormant imaginative spark deep within you and provide an opportunity for healing.

Getting Into Your Body and Out of Your Mind

Two things immediately happen when I tell people I am a belly dancer. First, they ask if I meant to say "ballet" dancer. Next, they glance at my belly and wonder if it isn't a little too large to be exposed in public. I gently inform them with a smile and a wink that this ancient dance form celebrates women of all body types, shapes, and ages.

At 42, I found myself at a health food store picking up acidophilus for my one-year-old, who had diarrhea due to antibiotic therapy. This was his second bout of antibiotics in the past six months, and his GI system was not happy. I felt like a walking zombie. My T-shirt was wrinkled and smelled like vomit from Robert, my three-year-old, who also had some stomach flu. I hadn't changed my sweatpants in days, and my hair was in a messy bun, best described as a bird's nest. With acidophilus, applesauce, and bananas in hand, I avoided eye contact with the check-out clerk and hoped he had a weak sense of smell. A small flyer on the counter area caught my eye as I grabbed my bag.

Who knew that this little flyer, no bigger than the palm of my hand, would change my life forever?

It featured a dancer with a big skirt and coin bra, arms open and confident, twirling with her head tilted slightly back. She wore a big smile, and several flowers adorned her hair. At that moment, dazed and waiting in line, she talked to me and let me know that I needed to join her six-week introductory tribal belly dance class starting the next month. The beaming dancer reassured me that no prior dance experience was required. She whispered a reminder of how much I used to love to go out dancing with my husband, an activity I had long since given up as part of the tradeoff to raise my kids and run a company.

Later that night, after dinner, I showed my husband, Kris, the pocket-sized flyer. "What do you think?" I asked.

"Go," he said without a second of hesitation.

"What about the kids?" I asked.

"I got them. No worries. You need to dance."

The day before the first class, I panicked. What was I going to wear? There was no way in hell I was going to expose my pillowy belly that had been stretched and rearranged to accommodate two recent children. A quick sweep of my closet for possible outfits was even more dismaying. All I had to choose from were professional dresses and suits or sweatpants and T-shirts. I looked at the flyer to see if there were any hints about what to wear. It stated, "Dress comfortably for movement."

I finally decided on navy sweatpants with pink fuchsia piping on either side and a matching long-sleeved, ribbed T-shirt. It was 6:40 p.m., and I was ready to kiss my husband and the kids goodbye and reassure them, "Mommy will be back soon." My one-year-old, Jackson, started crying.

"Go," my husband pleaded.

"I just can't," I said. Tears were in my eyes, too.

In a remarkable moment of determination, I stood up, landed Jackson in my husband's arms, and ran toward the door. I heard Jackson's wailing on the other side of the door, but I kept walking forward. I opened my car door, entered the driver's seat, and turned on the ignition.

Looking in the mirror to back out of the garage, I caught a glimpse of my reflection. My hair looked cute, with bangs and my usual bird's nest bun in the back. I had remembered to put on some lipstick. My mascara was running from the tears welling up in my eyes, but it didn't stop me. I drove to class that evening filled with a confluence of pure excitement and an intense yearning to reconnect with the girl inside who loved to dance and twirl. From deep within, an inner voice took charge and piloted me to exactly where I needed to go.

Many of us (that includes you) super-achieving scientific types have dedicated ourselves to our fields of study, and in doing so, we have left our original hobbies and artistic passions in the dust. Who can blame us? We had to finish college, pay bills, start the painful adulting process, and get laser-focused on succeeding in our field and proving ourselves. On top of that, you might be caring for others or burdened with a mountain of obligations, making it seem like you don't have time to engage your creativity.

Here is the simple truth. Now is the time to discover or reclaim the beautiful expanse of who you are, in addition to your daily job and life obligations. Even if you can only commit to engaging in creativity for a few minutes a week, it makes a difference. Stop thinking about all the reasons you can't do it, and instead, listen to that internal hum, get in the metaphorical car, turn on the ignition, and drive!

As Julie Cameron, author of *The Artist's Way*, suggests, "In filling the well of creativity, think magic. Think delight. Think fun. Do not think duty. Do not do what you should do—do what intrigues you."

The Benefits of Dancing for All Ages

At the age of 61, I still belly dance. I shimmy weekly with our troupe, ReBel-lyon, and teach classes on dance and body positivity at a local museum. On the next page is a photo of us backstage before a performance.

Our troupe delivers family-friendly performances at local fundraisers, dazzling audiences as we balance swords on our heads, play zills, and sashay across the floor in rhythm with the music. The women in our troupe range in age from 31 to 67. We are teachers, biology majors, PhDs, coffee shop managers, nurses, moms, wives, and a diabetes specialist. If you had told me on that day in the health food store that I would belly dance in public as part of a troupe for twenty years, I would have stared at you in sheer disbelief. But now I've realized a simple truth: I will never stop dancing again, not only because of the cardiovascular benefits or to maintain a smaller waistline. There are countless other, more important reasons I am committed to dancing for as long as possible.

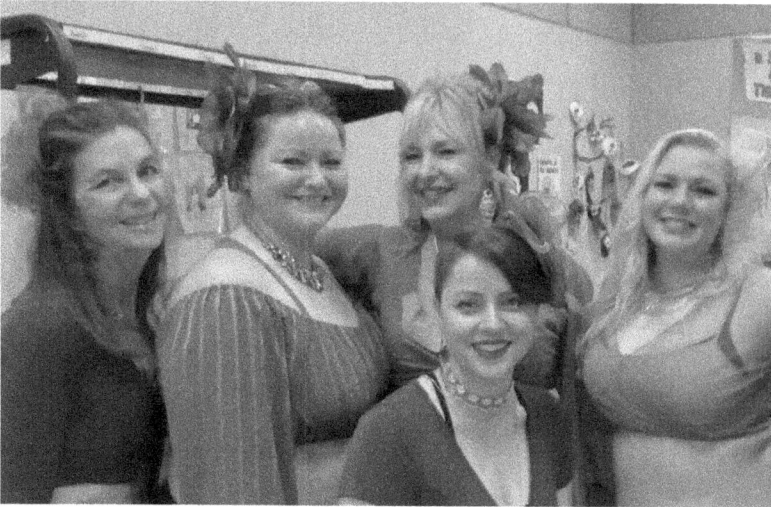

The year I started taking belly dance classes, I was halfway through writing a chapter for a nursing textbook on the relationship between cardiovascular disease and diabetes. I spent hours digging through research papers, trying to consolidate complicated information into understandable paragraphs. It was rough going, but it became noticeably easier when I started dancing. It seemed that asking my body to move in new ways and memorizing choreography was lighting up my brain. My writing flowed more naturally, making presenting scientific data in a clear, intelligible format easier. I was able to grasp how complex concepts interconnected and discern their underlying relationships more quickly.

In dance class, I had to work hard on getting my left non-dominant hand to participate in the choreography and make it look elegant. Little did I know that I was building a whole new neural freeway system in my brain while strengthening and connecting with my body.

The scientific data backs up my experience. Dancing significantly enhances neuroplasticity—the brain's ability to adapt and form new neural connections—due to its combination of physical movement, mental engagement, and emotional expression (Lavinia Teixeira-Machado et al., 2018). Learning dance steps in sequence engages memory and learning, creating new pathways and improving cognitive flexibility. Dancing integrates auditory, visual, and proprioceptive (body awareness) inputs. Given this multisensory experience, dancing enhances connections between different brain regions, fostering greater adaptability and efficiency (Fissler et al., 2018). Dancing also makes us feel good since it is associated with increased levels of dopamine, serotonin, and BDNF (Brain-Derived Neurotrophic Factor), which is essential for neuroplasticity (Rehfeld et al., 2018).

In addition to improving idea integration, dancing enhanced my confidence and made me a more dynamic and physical public speaker. I felt more comfortable moving around in my body and less self-conscious standing in the front of the class. Knowing how much dancing improved learning, I started leading dance moves during my lectures, encouraging the audience to stand up and join in. I would incorporate left and right body activities to activate both sides of participants' brains to help them assimilate content-dense topics. Attendees of my conferences learn the diabetes flash mob, the Macarena, and other body crossover moves. Humans are built for movement, and our brains function more effectively when we stay active.

Social dancing fosters human connection, which activates the social brain network and supports neuroplastic changes associated with empathy and communication. The simple act of getting the class up and dancing transforms a quiet audience into a laughing and connected group of movement enthusiasts.

Blending My Passions: Encouraging People with Diabetes to Dance

When we are least expecting it, the universe sends us instructions. I did not envision myself as a dancer or imagine that I would teach dance moves to healthcare professionals while presenting at diabetes conferences. By blending my passion with my profession, I found a more profound sense of authenticity, embracing all parts of myself while encouraging others to do the same.

Inspired by how dancing revitalized and engaged professionals, I started incorporating it into classes I taught for individuals living with diabetes. Enhancing neuroplasticity is especially beneficial for people with diabetes, as they face a significantly higher risk of developing dementia due to elevated or low blood glucose levels and other related factors. Regular dancing reduces cognitive decline and improves memory in aging brains. By combining physical, mental, and emotional elements, dancing uniquely stimulates the brain, fostering resilience and adaptability, all while improving balance. Of course, we must consider our audience and be cognizant of limitations and physical safety. With the easy availability of YouTube, there is now access to all levels of dance movement instructions that match the individual's ability. I encourage people to explore styles and music that resonate with them and start slowly.

If dancing isn't your thing, there are plenty of other creative activities to explore—gardening, yoga, tai chi, Zumba, or organized sports like Pickleball all offer similar benefits. Dancing is one example of how hobbies that engage our creativity while incorporating body movement can enrich our lives. It highlights the importance of honoring creativity as a vital part of life, even if we're initially unsure of its value.

Ideas to Light Your Creative Spark

Did you have a childhood or adult hobby you loved doing? One that made you lose track of time as you entered the zone referred to as "flow"? Have you given yourself permission to make time for that hobby and lose yourself in that creative process? You may want to take a ceramics or writing class, join the local choir, or start a band. Perhaps you found an old camera and want to learn more about photography or realized you're good at painting. It can be hard to start as a beginner and potentially look silly or unskilled. Here's my advice: Let go of those sky-high expectations. No one expects you to paint like Monet in your first art class. My motto is, if something makes me uncomfortable, I know I'm in the right place—because that's where growth happens. I encourage you to take that leap of faith and tolerate the momentary discomfort for long-term gain. It gets better, and before you know it, you will blossom in ways you never expected.

Here is a list of 20 creative endeavors that you might consider pursuing. You may already be doing one or more of these, or you may have new ideas to add to the list. Fantastic; keep up the great work!

20 Creative Endeavors to Consider

Painting

Writing poetry or fiction

Playing a musical instrument

Photography

Sculpting or pottery

Dancing

Singing or songwriting

Acting, theater performance, and improvisation

Graphic design or digital art

Cooking or baking creatively

Crafting (e.g., knitting, crocheting, quilting)

Interior design or home decoration

Journaling or bullet journaling

Filmmaking or video editing

Gardening or landscaping

Calligraphy or hand lettering

Designing jewelry or accessories

Building models or DIY projects

Woodworking or carpentry

Creating comic strips or animations

Closet Creatives: Acknowledging Your Creativity Without Shame

I didn't know purple was my favorite color until I was in my forties. I thought that being successful meant I had to block out all that creative stuff and focus on growing my company and being an attentive mom and partner. After five years of building my business, raising a family, and belly dancing, I proclaimed after a dance performance pictured here, "I am an artist." My husband laughed and said, "I thought you were a Diabetes Specialist?" I thought for a minute and replied, "I am a Diabetes Specialist who sees the world through an artist's lens." Here is a photo of me, taken by Jony Weiss, dancing at our local museum as part of a fund-raising campaign.

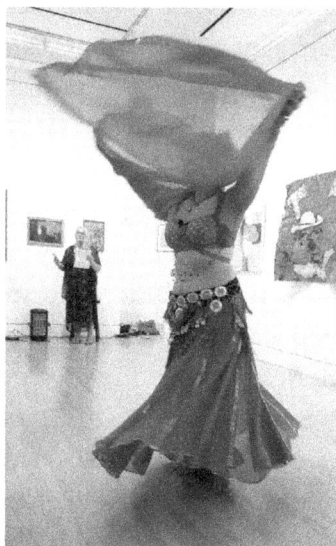

Dancing has allowed me to see myself as a nurse and a performance artist. This was a turning point in my life. By proclaiming the truth of who I am out loud, I finally recognized the importance of my artistic and scientific selves. I also realized they could stand side-by-side, holding hands while sharing the most intimate details of their latest discoveries. This newly revealed integration allowed me to express myself with more complexity and authenticity in my personal and professional life, and it felt great!

There was a brief period of cognitive dissonance as the integration began to take hold, starting with my clothes. Little by little, my belly dancing colors seeped into my closet, and my clothes began taking on a lavender hue. Slowly, my professional wardrobe went from mainly black formal suit jackets and pencil skirts to brightly colored flowery outfits that flounced when walking. My scientific professional side questioned if my clothes were too outlandish and wild; after all, I was a professional speaker. My artistic side gently nudged me toward a fresh, sparkly authenticity that included lots of bling, maroon highlights, hair flowers, and increased vulnerability. I was worried about rejection and push-back from my colleagues, but they loved this fun look and encouraged me to keep dressing like "I was going to a party."

This commitment to authentic expression made me a more effective and engaging presenter to whom my audience could relate. I incorporated more storytelling and human experiences along with evidence-based information. More professionals enrolled in my online classes and asked me to speak at their diabetes continuing education events.

The universe was delivering a clear message: Stepping into my most authentic self unlocked the best version of me. More than that, it gave other people permission to move toward authenticity, too.

A diabetes dietitian colleague and close friend, whose house burned down in the 2019 Camp Fire, has been writing "morning pages" for half an hour every day as encouraged in Julia Cameron's classic book, *The Artist's Way*. My friend has been searching for a way to honor her dietitian expertise and heal from her trauma while incorporating her love of food and cooking artistry. During a recent breakfast date, her face lit up with complete joy as she described her idea for a new business that came to her during her morning writing. She wants to start a small business to cook soups and healthy meals for her healthcare professional colleagues, blending her nutrition expertise and love into every dish.

Have you dreamed about ways to combine your passion with your profession? Or have you even considered changing careers to turn your passion into profit? By allowing yourself to explore these thoughts and even actualize them, you are sending a strong message to that playful and creative inner being that they are seen and heard. Sometimes, that simple acknowledgment may be the start of something magical.

Pursuing Creative Passions Helps Heal Trauma

As a healthcare professional, you are well-versed in hearing and witnessing trauma, and you may be holding your own trauma stories. I mentioned earlier that belly dancing changed my life forever. I might even go as far as to say it saved my life.

When people think of belly dancing, it may conjure up images of a bewitching woman in a glamorous outfit shaking her hips (and other body parts) in a Middle Eastern restaurant. When I think of belly dancing, it conjures respect for a centuries-old dance form passed on from mother to daughter. In contrast to popular belief, belly dancing was not performed for men.

Traditionally, belly dancing was performed in spaces where women gathered away from men. Today, many women consider belly dancing a fun and therapeutic activity, reconnecting them with their bodies and fostering emotional well-being and body positivity. By dancing together, women affirm their identities, share their struggles, and enjoy a sense of empowerment.

Dancing with my sisters not only allowed me to express my artistry but also opened the door to begin healing from my childhood trauma. It allowed me to reclaim my body and be grounded in its power and sensuality. This art form became a sanctuary—a space where I could twirl, shake my shaker, and move freely, without shame or judgment, fully embracing the joy of my life at that moment.

Creative pursuits are potent tools in the healing process for healthcare professionals and those who have survived trauma. By fostering self-expression, enhancing emotional regulation, and creating opportunities for connection, they can be a source of comfort and relief. As you heal and become more regulated, you will likely become more present at your job, home, and community. There will be more space for self-compassion and expanded grace for yourself and others.

In addition to healthcare professionals, people living with diabetes often carry a history of trauma and pain that can add to the complexity of managing a very demanding chronic condition. Encouraging them to tap into their creativity can offer a respite and provide an opportunity to rediscover a long-lost passion or the joys of a newfound hobby, which can be especially helpful as part of their overall diabetes management plan.

Yet, finding a hobby is not enough for you or those with diabetes to heal. Even though I was honoring my need for self-expression and creativity, there was a deeper, hidden part of me that I kept ignoring and pushing aside. This shadow part, carved from past painful experiences, needed healing and attention. Like many healthcare professionals, I had been so focused on caring for my family and running my company that I failed to heed the warning signs my own body was sending me.

• • •

The next chapter reveals how two unexpected health crises forced me to pause, confront what I had long ignored, and ultimately reshape the path toward my future self. These health events weren't simply obstacles—they became the turning points that redefined my understanding of resilience, self-care, and the intricate connection between mind, body, and purpose.

CHAPTER 7

The Body Tells the Story

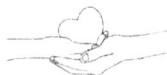

"There is no greater agony than bearing an untold story inside you."

— Maya Angelou

At 53, I was on top of the world. My company was flourishing, my two boys, ages 10 and 12, were thriving, and my marriage was solid. Life felt like a joyful dance, each step in tune with the rhythm of my growing responsibilities and an unshakable positive outlook. But beneath the surface, the cracks in my foundation were intensifying. Little did I know that I was about to be dealt the first of many blows that would force me to come to terms with the emotional trauma of my childhood that I thought I had left far behind.

It started out as an ordinary morning, rushing to get the kids ready for school, preparing breakfast, and writing my to-do list for the day. But something was wrong. The words on the paper did not match the words in my head. I slurped down my coffee to see if a fast dose of caffeine would clear the cobwebs and tried to yell for the kids to, "Come get breakfast." But I couldn't assign the right words to my instructions. Instead, I called breakfast butter. I asked them if they wanted milk on their toast. I stammered my words. I stood in the middle of the kitchen and cried. Then I whispered, "I think I am having a stroke."

My 12-year-old son Robert grabbed his cell phone and called my husband, who was working as a pharmacist at a nearby hospital. Kris directed Robert to, "Call 911 NOW."

I grabbed Robert's phone and reassured my husband that I was fine and did not need an ambulance. I hung up and hustled my kids into the car, worried they would be late for school. As I drove them to their different schools, I provided a detailed summary of all the recent news events I could remember to prove I was okay. After all, I was only 53 and healthy.

During that 20-minute kid drop-off route, my husband called me at least six times until I finally picked up the phone. He commanded, "Get your ass to the hospital NOW!" The entire stroke team was waiting for me.

I finally relented, and at 8:47 a.m. on a blue-sky Wednesday morning, I was in the emergency room. The stroke team started their familiar choreography. They rushed me into a gown, hooked up monitors, drew blood, and laid me on the gurney for a CT scan of the brain. The results came back fast. There was no bleeding in the brain; it was a non-hemorrhagic event, and I had no lingering stroke symptoms that I knew of.

Three hours after the event, I was ready to go home. Convinced this was all a mistake since my CT scan, labs, and heart rhythm looked good, I questioned why I should waste precious hospital resources with an overnight stay. The team insisted I stay and wait for the results of the MRI of my brain, scheduled for the next morning. I spent the night in the hospital, getting neuro checks every four hours, playing with the controls on my bed, and keeping a brave face when I told shocked family members and friends of the series of events.

Truth be told, for the past 30 years, I have been fighting for my life and my health. My dad suffered a heart attack at 39 and a stroke at 44. He died a month after his 56th birthday, a month short of meeting his future son-in-law and ten years short of taking his grandkids out to play ball. His shortened life was a central motivating force for my healthy lifestyle.

To guarantee my health, I walked 55 miles a week, taught belly dance classes, and ate a diet filled with vegetables, fruit, fiber, and an occasional glass of red wine. My lifestyle habits put me at low risk for stroke, but my genetics worked against me.

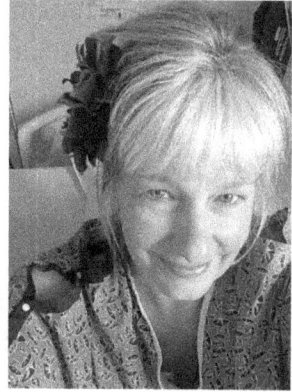

I was up at 6:30 a.m. the following day, mentally ready to get discharged from the hospital. I decided to try some dance choreography in my room to see if I could remember the sequence of moves. My balance was off-kilter, and I felt nauseated after some spins, but I chalked that up to lack of sleep. I wrapped my hair in a bun with two bobby pins that I found at the bottom of my purse. To show everyone I would be okay, I clipped a big fuchsia flower above my ear as pictured.

At 11 a.m., the technician rolled me into the noisy, rhythmic banging tunnel of the MRI machine. I imagined the magnetic energy exploring the nooks, crannies, and undulations of my white matter, searching for injured brain tissue—an exploration I was sure would turn up empty-handed.

At 12:40 p.m., the neurologist walked into the room, saying he had read the results of my MRI and explained that I had suffered a stroke in the Wernicke or language comprehension center of my brain. What he said after that, I don't remember.

He left the room, and a flood of tears started pouring from my eyes. My husband, who was working in the hospital, flew into the room, breathless from running up three flights of stairs after I texted him to "please come." He saw my distress and wrapped me in his arms. He whispered a sweet Armenian prayer, blessing me and asking for God's healing powers.

Despite this setback, I felt great, except for a nagging pain in my right leg, and quickly returned to running my company, walking three-four hours daily on my treadmill desk. My 12-year-old son wrote me the most touching birthday card a few weeks afterward. He wrote, "Mom, you taught me that it's not what happens to you but how you bounce back." Yet, since that day, I have been a slightly different version of myself. If you met me on the street or at a conference, you probably would have no clue about my stroke history. And, according to my family, I am pretty much the same as before. But I can't pretend that the stroke didn't leave its mark. Sometimes, I need to try harder to remember or say words correctly. Occasionally, I blurt out a word that doesn't yet exist. But sometimes, I feel like I can express myself even better.

At the time, I considered this event "my stroke of luck"—an early warning sign that forced me to take action to prevent a more debilitating stroke. Up to this point in my life, I had only seen this stroke event through the lens of science, as a vascular defect that resulted from the lousy genes my dad passed on to me. Now, I share my stroke signs and the importance of early intervention with my community to increase awareness and hopefully save future lives.

Learning to Stay Attuned to Your Body Messages

As a healthcare professional, you likely turn your focus outward, caring for others ahead of yourself, almost as if this quality is infused into the Hippocratic oath. I can't count how many times I have seen my husband arrive home completely spent after working ten hours trying to keep critically ill people alive. My close friend, a counselor who bears witness to the trauma of first responders and leads debriefings to help people process unbearable tragedy, arrives at our book club completely exhausted. On top of your work duties, you may have children or parents to care for and check in with, coupled with the responsibilities of paying bills and keeping your household running.

This giving of self and tending to others may leave you too depleted to check in with yourself or look under the hood to see if everything is still running smoothly or if a tune-up is required. This state of busyness can also act as a shelter to shield yourself from addressing those hard feelings that have been pushed aside or buried deep within. Our bodies send us signals through gastrointestinal distress, headaches, flare-ups of autoimmune conditions, or even cardiovascular disease. You may have noticed your body giving you messages that everything was not right, but you may have brushed it off since you didn't have any resources to allocate for yourself.

According to the Mortality and Morbidity World Report, people who have experienced significant childhood trauma have double the risk of experiencing a heart attack or stroke. After my ischemic event, despite running every kind of test, probing my heart for defects, and testing for arrhythmias with various heart monitors, the doctors could not discover the cause of my ischemic stroke. The event was deemed cryptogenic, which in Latin means "of obscure or unknown origin." My body was warning me that something was out of balance and needed attention and care. Instead of slowing down and giving space for healing, I was angry at this betrayal and fired up to prove my body wrong. As quoted from *The Body Keeps the Score* by Bessel van der Kolk, "As long as you keep secrets and suppress information, you are fundamentally at war with yourself. The critical issue is allowing yourself to know what you know."

This wasn't the last of my body sending me messages I chose not to hear. Within days of being discharged from the hospital, I was back at my desk, directing the choir of my life as if nothing had happened. I felt overjoyed that I had cheated death, and my mental capacity still felt as sharp as ever. But I did have this nagging right foot and leg pain that seemed to get worse with each passing day until I finally drove myself to urgent care to make sure my foot wasn't broken. The X-ray revealed that all bones were in proper alignment without any fractures. But the icy-hot burning pain persisted, worsening at night or if I stood on my feet without moving for too long. I mentioned this new pain at my neurologist's follow-up appointment, and he probed my nerves with electrical stimulation to make sure they were intact and firing. My leg nerves registered healthy, and then an 'aha' look flashed across his face, and he quietly said, almost to himself, "Thalamic pain syndrome." He wrote me a prescription for my nerve pain and scheduled a follow-up appointment in a couple of weeks.

As soon as I was in the safety of my car, I Googled Thalamic Pain Syndrome, and Wikipedia filled me in on this new, angry friend who wouldn't seem to let go of my right leg. The description read, "an unfortunate outcome following a cerebrovascular accident (CVA). The pain experienced by the patient is centralized, neuropathic, and associated with temperature changes. Patients will often suffer from hyperalgesia (abnormally heightened sensitivity to pain) and allodynia (pain due to a stimulus that does not normally elicit pain). It is also known as central post-stroke pain syndrome and affects about 8% of all individuals post-stroke." Yes, this perfectly described this altered version of myself, and I realized I did not get off Scot-free after all.

Mourning the Loss of How You See Yourself

To my friends and colleagues reading these words, I want to share with complete honesty what happened next. The more I discovered about this poorly understood condition and the lack of effective treatment, the more I was consumed by anger, sorrow, and grief. I wasn't just suffering from the physical pain; I was hurting from the fundamental shift in how I perceived myself. These strong emotions translated into more pain and burning in my affected leg. I couldn't understand why this happened to me. For weeks, I ugly cried and raised my tear-filled eyes to the sky, begging for an answer.

With time and the unconditional support of my husband, kids, and friends, this storm of grief dissipated and slowly turned into a breeze of reluctant acceptance. Not willing to take opiates or mood-altering medications, I had to find other ways to soothe my pain and bring my body into calmness. The first step was accepting this clingy, chronic hurt and asking it what it needed to feel comforted and cared for. The touch of my husband's hands holding my foot, warm baths, reading a great book, hanging out with friends, dancing, and walking became the remedies I turned to that brought comfort to my leg and were a healing salve to my emotional despair.

I was also able to move on from the initial isolation that my new condition brought me. I thought about all the people I serve with diabetes who also suffer from peripheral neuropathy, or friends and family who have chronic back, knee, or hip pain. People with arthritis and joint inflammation, sports injuries, and other disabilities. I was not alone in my suffering, and even more, my pain increased my empathy with others who face physical limitations and chronic pain. Experiencing this firsthand made me more attuned to the struggles that often go unnoticed and more committed to finding ways to recognize and alleviate the pain many people silently endure.

However, even with all this growth, I still wasn't ready to address the emotional roots of my physical pain.

Over the next five years, I became an expert at dodging my leg pain and pushing it into the background. Determined not to let it slow me down, I kept taking on new challenges, growing my company, and moving my life forward. I led our dance troupe and attended my kids' basketball games, chess matches, and musical performances. My husband and boys, Robert and Jackson, pictured on the next page, decided we needed to start adventuring. We traipsed through Croatia, spent four weeks camping in national parks, and played

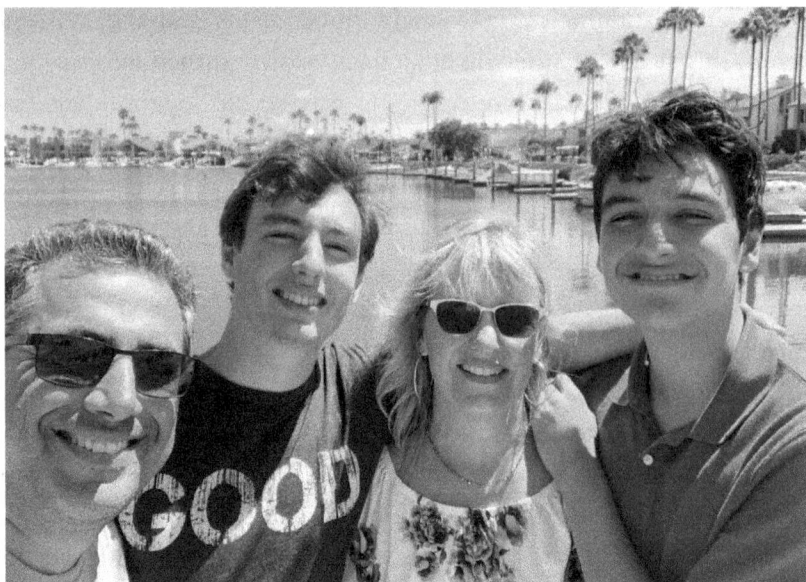

highly competitive card games in our Airstream trailer. But there was still something inside of me that was not quite right; a nagging dark shadow that would find me during quiet moments when I was still and not distracted by the activities of my life.

Your Body Holds the Memory

December and January are always my busiest times of the year, when, besides doing all the usual stuff for the holiday season, my business is in full swing, updating our entire library of online courses to reflect the yearly American Diabetes Association standards. It is a demanding time for my entire team, and we need all hands on deck to pull this miracle off. Even when things are running in perfect rhythm, I still work many extra hours to ensure my first quarter's two dozen courses reflect the latest science and evidence.

Amid this crazy time, my full-time operations manager gave me her two weeks' notice in a letter left on my desk over the New Year's holiday. The job was not a good match for her, and I understood why she was leaving, but the timing could not have been worse. Somewhere deep inside of me, this notice of quitting triggered feelings of abandonment that had long since been dormant.

Later that night, hanging out with my family, I began experiencing intense palpitations and irregular heartbeats. Throughout menopause, my heart would act up on a regular basis, but this episode was unrelenting and especially nerve-racking. I tried everything to stop them, including deep breathing, meditation, dancing, drinking water, watching reels with my kids, and bearing down. Nothing was working, so we decided to head to the emergency room. In the intake room, they hooked me up to an EKG and verified I was having plenty of PVCs and my blood pressure was elevated. The next moment, my feelings of panic melted away, and I felt utterly relaxed. So relaxed that I purposely slid off the chair and onto the emergency room floor to get more comfortable.

Thinking about it now, I want to cry-laugh at my husband's simultaneously shocked and panicked face. His wife, the mother of his children and CEO of a company, was sitting on the hospital floor like she was enjoying a picnic at a park. He looked at the staff and said, "This is a definite change." They lifted me up, whisked me onto a gurney, and paged the neurologist on call "stat." He asked me a dizzying barrage of questions and expected me to answer them immediately. The neurologist didn't seem to recognize that I had downshifted into a recently discovered slow gear in my brain that could not keep up with him.

If you have ever met me or heard me lecture, you will know that this is the complete antithesis of everything about me. I am all about motion and forward movement. But on this gurney, underneath bright fluorescent lights, I couldn't figure out why everyone was in such a rush. On top of speaking more haltingly than Barack Obama, I was cursing like a sailor. I hadn't dropped that many "F" bombs since college. This was particularly shocking to me since, as a trained and disciplined healthcare professional, I would never use swear words when conferring with my colleagues. I kept apologizing to the neurologist, who nodded in understanding, but my mouth kept uttering a litany of profanity without regard to the audience.

I was admitted to the neuro floor with the diagnosis of epileptic seizures and started on anti-seizure medications.

The seizures continued despite the medications. I would suddenly downshift to slow gear, start crying, and repeat over and over that, "I didn't feel good" or that I was "a loser." The nurses would sit with me during these episodes, hold my hand, and give me tissues. They reassured me that I was not a loser. They were angels who loved and protected this broken little soul, trying to find her way. When I woke up scared one night, they moved me right next to the nurse's station so I would feel safe. They intuitively knew what I needed, and I felt blanketed in their nurturing.

By the fifth hospital day, my seizures had not stopped. The new neurologist on-call assessed me and immediately insisted I be transferred to a teaching hospital with 24-hour camera monitoring and continuous EEG to verify that these seizures were epileptic in origin. After two days of close observation, the medical team entered my room and delivered a new diagnosis. I was not experiencing epileptic seizures emanating from crossed circuits in the brain. Based on the EEGs and their observation, I was experiencing psychogenic seizures resulting from emotional trauma.

These experts explained that high-functioning, super-achieving individuals can suffer from psychogenic seizures, often as a result of unprocessed physical, emotional, or sexual abuse during childhood. Psychogenic Non-Epileptic Seizures (PNES) are the body's physical expression of unresolved trauma. They are not a reflection of weakness or failure but a complex interplay between the mind and body reaching a breaking point. Hearing this was both a relief and a challenge. On the one hand, it gave me a framework to understand what was happening, but on the other, it forced me to finally confront the emotional pain I had kept hidden safely away for so long.

A Note to the Reader

Thank you for sitting with me through the telling of this very personal and painful story. A frightened part of me wants to keep this part hidden because it is so tender and vulnerable. The part of me that craves validation wants you to see me as someone who has it all together, confident, unstoppable, and ready to conquer anything that comes my way.

However, I chose to risk sharing my story to liberate myself—and anyone else who needs to hear it—from the weight of shame that has burdened many of us for far too long. Shame thrives in secrecy but bringing it into the open through self-reflection or connection with others can loosen its grip and lead to healing. Like me, maybe your body has been trying to send you gentle messages urging you to unwrap the package of pain or shame that may be tucked away for safety. Over time, these unattended signals can wreak havoc on your body. Maybe it is time to attend to this injured bird and give it wings to fly and reclaim its place in this world.

As Mary Oliver wisely writes in her famous poem "Wild Geese," "You do not have to be good. You do not have to walk on your knees for a hundred miles through the desert, repenting. You only have to let the soft animal of your body love what it loves."

Moving Toward Healing

The day after I was discharged from the hospital, I called a local mental health counselor and asked for help. He listened carefully to my story, paused, and said, "I can hold your pain and help you on this journey." Through a combination of intensive therapy using Internal Family Systems or "Family parts therapy," an approach developed by psychologist Richard Schwartz, cognitive behavioral therapy, journaling, dancing, and the unrelenting support of my gracious husband, children, and friends, I am healing. The shadow that once lingered in hidden corners now shows itself far less often. Occasionally, I still grapple with PTSD and waves of intense shame and failure, but these moments are no longer buried in secrecy. Instead, I bring them into the open, sharing them with my husband and close friends. By naming my shame and exposing it to the light, I release myself from the weight of self-judgment, allowing my bird spirit to once again soar free.

As a caregiver who may have suffered trauma or abuse yourself, I encourage you to take time to shine the light of healing from within. To give space to discover that voice in you that knows what is needed to regulate and integrate yourself as a beautiful being, whether through hobbies, art, music, therapy, or an alternative healing path. As you gift yourself space for healing, you also have a heightened capacity to connect with your friends, family, and the people you serve. And through this shared humanity, there is an opportunity to create a bridge where healing flows both ways.

• • •

The next chapter will take you on a deep dive into the importance of taking time for your own healing and well-being. Trust me, there is no mention of eating enough high-fiber foods or the importance of staying active. However, there are plenty of fresh approaches to gifting yourself the kindness and self-compassion you so thoroughly deserve.

CHAPTER 8

Healing the Healer

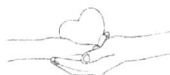

"The work of healing requires that we bring our full selves—messy, tired, hopeful, broken, and brave—to the table."

— adrienne maree brown

"Mom, you should try mushrooms," my 19-year-old practically yelled as we watched the documentary *Fantastic Fungi*. As a chemistry major, he was riveted by the film we were watching. It explored the therapeutic uses of mushrooms, especially psilocybin, for their potential to address not only mental health issues but also physical ailments such as neuropathy.

I laughed and replied, "Me? I've never done anything stronger than pot, and that was more than 30 years ago." But as I went to bed that night, something unexpected stirred within me—a feeling I hadn't allowed myself to entertain when it came to my chronic nerve pain.

It was a feeling of hope.

Over the next 12 months, I immersed myself in learning about the therapeutic use of this ancient medicine. I listened to podcasts, devoured books and articles by leading experts, and explored the latest research on using a single dose of psilocybin to treat nerve pain.

After seven years of trying everything—from electrical stimulation to creams, medications, and CBD gummies—I was more than ready to find relief from the relentless icy-burning sensation that haunted my right leg and foot.

Countless discussions with my husband and friends about the pros and cons led to the final decision—move forward. I began researching safe and legal locations outside of California that offered psilocybin therapy and signed up for my first experience at a certified center in Oregon. I packed up my family, and we made the four-hour trip north.

Preparing for a psilocybin experience involves setting a clear intention and being open to letting go of control or ego, allowing the medicine to guide you. I arrived at the clinic with a bag of mementos, including a picture of my family, a heart-shaped crystal, and a photo of my aunt. I clutched my intention of "healing my nerves and allowing for less inflammation throughout my body," written on bright pink paper.

My guide, Carmen, was a retired physician with extensive knowledge of guiding people on psilocybin. She welcomed me with a hug and explained how she had prepared the room to be free of negative spirits by burning sage and blessing the space. As we got ready, her presence calmed me. I knew her safekeeping and oversight would protect me during the journey. I set up an altar on the table with my mementos and pictures. I propped up my pink papered intention on my aunt's photo frame and felt ready for whatever came next.

Carmen brought in the hot water and dried mushroom powder. She instructed me on how to make the tea. I added honey to the warm mushroom beverage and drank the entire cup. I settled onto the couch and listened to a recorded meditation by a researcher from the Johns Hopkins Institute. Her soothing voice and the music gently carried me into an underwater ocean, inviting me to explore what the medicine wished to reveal.

By the time the meditation stopped, the magic of the mushrooms kicked in. A galaxy of lights appeared against a deep blue sky, and in a rainbow of colors, Alex and Ying, my beloved adopted family from Ying's Chinese Restaurant, welcomed me. I cried tears of joy for this reunion, and, of course, I proudly counted from one to twenty in Cantonese to let them know I hadn't forgotten. They laughed and encouraged me to keep moving forward since a cherished guide awaited me. In the next unexpected moment, my dad, who had died from a sudden heart attack over 25 years ago, stood there before me. (Here is a photo of me and my dad, the last time I saw him alive, when I was 35.)

I gasped and said, "Dad, I thought you had forgotten me."

"No." He nodded. "Do you know how hard I've been working to connect with you?"

My dad and I sat amongst the stars for the next two hours and talked. I shared the anger from my trauma and detailed how it had impacted me. I told him about his son-in-law and his grandkids, whom he had never had the chance to meet. We finally got to have our father-daughter wedding dance, and then we said goodbye. I remember asking him if he could check with his doctors on the "other side" to see if they had any remedies for nerve pain, and he promised he would.

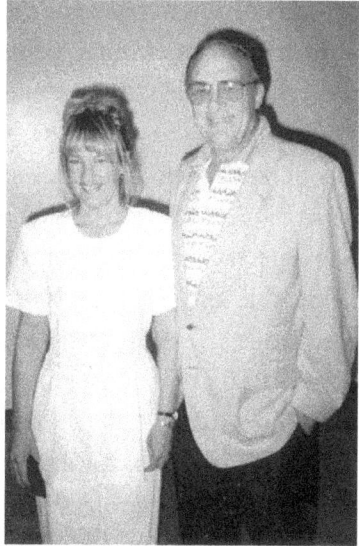

As I continue to unpack this life-changing experience, I keep receiving an abundance of unexpected gifts from this plant medicine. Besides having the opportunity to share my truth with my dad, my anxiety and "loop" thinking diminished. My ability to speak Spanish and word recall improved, and I began considering situations from fresh perspectives. I felt more integrated and whole. Those feelings have not diminished. They've deepened over time, becoming a quiet but steady source of clarity, connection, and inner strength.

These effects aren't just a placebo. Research published in the journal *Nature* used brain imaging techniques, like MRI, to show that the brain enters a state of heightened plasticity under the influence of psilocybin. This means that previously unconnected regions of the brain start communicating more freely. These new connections can lead to fresh perspectives, novel insights, and a sense of mental clarity. This rewiring is thought to underlie the reported improvements in emotional well-being and the ability to approach problems from a different, often healthier, perspective. Equally important is psilocybin's ability to weaken old neural connections that no longer serve us—those tied to deeply ingrained negative thought patterns or traumatic memories. By reducing these unhelpful connections, psilocybin creates space for new, healthier patterns to take root.

In alignment with the research findings, I am better able to recognize authentic feelings since they don't get lost in a maze of well-worn thought patterns. Even though my leg pain did not diminish, I am more at peace with it. I feel energized in my work and more willing to be vulnerable and honest with my struggles. This experience moved me forward in my emotional health in areas where I was genuinely stuck, despite years of counseling. My therapist was thrilled with my growth and ability to shed old thinking patterns. And if you are wondering if I would do it again, the answer is yes.

My goal in sharing this unfiltered story is to offer a message of hope for healing and to inspire you to take that bold, transformative step forward—whatever that may look like for you—starting today.

Getting to Your Best Mindbody Health

I am going to suggest something completely outlandish. I urge you to prioritize your mental and physical well-being in ways you haven't allowed yourself to. I am not suggesting that you sign up for psilocybin therapy (well, not yet anyway). But I implore you to take intentional steps to nurture and care for yourself, whether through getting enough sleep, connecting with loved ones, allowing yourself moments of stillness, or expressing your most authentic self. By prioritizing your well-being, you protect your energy and role model the importance of self-care, creating more balance and resilience in your life.

The hope is that replenishing your energy and nurturing your mindbody will create space for new opportunities and a more profound sense of fulfillment—because a rich, meaningful life is something you deserve!

Before we move on, you'll notice that I use the term "mindbody" as a single, unhyphenated word. This is intentional. It reflects a growing understanding among thought leaders that the mind and body are not separate systems, but one deeply interconnected whole. The term mindbody more accurately captures the dynamic relationship between our mental and physical selves, where thoughts, emotions, beliefs, and behaviors directly influence physical health, and the condition of the body, in turn, affects mental and emotional well-being.

As you explore this content, I invite you to reflect on practices that support and strengthen your mindbody connection. The advice in this chapter is not designed to add another activity to your already daunting to-do list. It is meant as a gift of healing and an opportunity to explore new ways of approaching your life and connecting more deeply with your authentic self.

Giving Yourself the Gift of Sleep

I used to wear my lack of sleep as a badge of honor. My motto was, "I'll have plenty of time to sleep when I am dead." I hastily dropped that motto after almost dying from a stroke. I know you have probably heard about sleep's benefits–how it improves cognition, enhances brain neuroplasticity, and helps with problem-solving and high performance. Getting adequate sleep keeps your gut bacteria happy (they need rest too) and decreases hunger hormones. It improves athletic performance, prevents cardiovascular disease, and gives you the stamina to make it over the finish line.

Yet, according to a study published at USC, the percentage of Americans reporting less than six hours of sleep a night increased from 29% to 33% from 2013 to 2017. The author, Jennifer Ailshire, says, "Poor sleep is a canary in a coal mine. We will see worse health outcomes as a result, and we may be seeing that already."

In a 2023 Gallup poll, 57% of Americans said they would feel better if they got more sleep, while 42% said they get enough sleep. Women are at higher risk of being underslept. Only 36% of women versus 48% of men say they get the sleep they need. Stress levels consistently contribute to a lack of sleep, and women experiencing stress have outpaced men by almost 10% over the past two decades. The relationship between stress and sleep is tightly interconnected. Stress contributes to less sleep, and not getting enough sleep can lead to higher levels of stress, along with frustration, depression, and anxiety. Sleep deprivation can also make it harder to cope with stressors and impact your ability to perceive the world accurately.

There are multitudes of books and articles about how to get more sleep, including descriptions of sleep hygiene habits such as turning off your phone, not having TVs in your bedroom, and trying to sleep at the same time every night, but sometimes it's hard to disconnect.

As a healthcare professional with competing demands and an emotionally taxing job, sleep is a gift your mindbody craves. If you struggle to get enough sleep without judgment, take a moment to envision one day in your life after getting enough sleep. How do you feel in your body and mind? What are you able to accomplish? How are your coping skills and ability to take on new challenges? Then, consider one step you might take to gift yourself an extra 15 minutes (or more) of sleep. Imagine that one step clearly or jot it down on a piece of paper or in your phone. Take a moment to consider how truly precious you are and all the people you help in your professional and personal life. You deserve this gift of sleep.

The Healing Power of Community

Our monthly Diabetes Support Group at a community hospital began with a handful of participants and eventually grew into a close-knit group of over thirty. We shared stories of triumph, compared blood glucose numbers, grieved losses, and celebrated joys—from white elephant gift exchanges to our annual Walk for Diabetes.

Over 15 years, the group naturally evolved as members started actively supporting each other, welcoming newcomers, answering questions, and providing encouragement through life's challenges. I was no longer needed to guide every moment; instead, I could step back and hold space for the healing already unfolding. This support group became a chosen family for them and me. But in 2018, everything changed. When the Camp Fire burned through Paradise, it destroyed our hospital and scattered the members across the country. The group was lost in the ashes, and with it, a cherished part of our lives.

Even though we no longer gather in the same room, the impact of those years still lives within us. The sense of connection we created—through consistency, vulnerability, and presence—remains a source of comfort and strength.

A more personal kind of connection unfolded when my two boys started junior high. I felt the window of time open up in my life. In that quiet shift, I realized how much I missed hanging out with girlfriends. So, we started the "No Guilt" Book Club—a space with a straightforward rule: Show up on the last Thursday of the month, whether or not you've read a single page.

For over a decade now, this group of women has gathered to share the deepest currents of our lives. We've held space for one another through the loss of parents, the unraveling of relationships, health scares, and the growing pains of raising children. What began as friends connecting quickly became a sacred circle—with plenty of laughter and tears. A safe place to share uncomfortable feelings, be vulnerable, and let go of saying the right thing. Through every chapter of life (and every half-read book), our "No Guilt" club has weathered storms and celebrated joy, including my 60th birthday, as pictured below. What a powerful reminder that simply showing up for each other, just as we are, is deeply healing. I know I can reach out to any of these amazing women and ask for help. They would be there for me and my family without hesitation, and I would do the same for them.

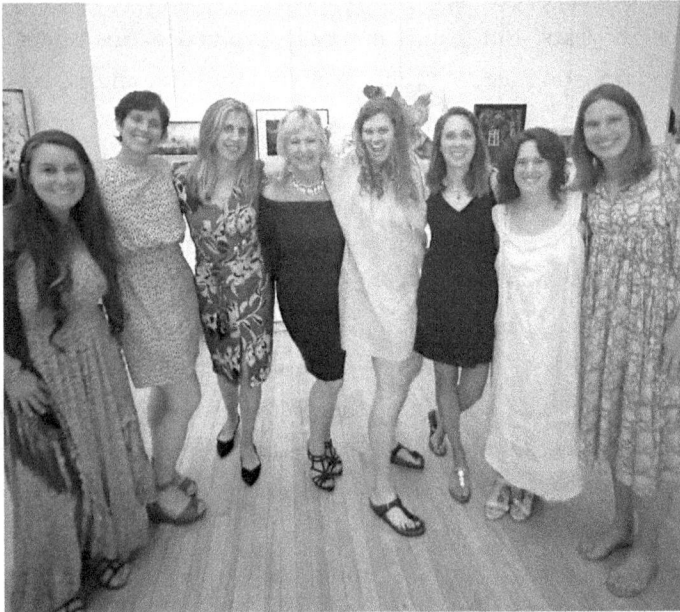

As Jane Howard once wrote, "Call it a clan, call it a network, call it a tribe, call it a family. Whatever you call it, whoever you are, you need one. You need one because you are human." Research backs this up. While the number of social groups needed for health varies by individual, studies suggest that belonging to three to five social groups significantly improves physical, mental, and emotional well-being. When one group becomes less accessible or supportive, others can help fill the gap, offering stability, perspective, and purpose.

Being part of a community is a vital part of being human. Social connection reduces stress, improves immune function, is associated with lower rates of depression, and even increases longevity.

Think for a moment about the groups you're part of:

- Family connections
- Close friendships
- Professional or workplace networks
- Community or hobby groups (clubs, volunteer work, faith communities)
- Health-focused groups (exercise or support groups)

Have you considered joining a group but felt hesitant or unsure whether you can commit the time and energy? That's completely understandable. Giving yourself permission to tune into what you need most, whether that's connection, rest, or something in between, is an essential part of caring for yourself. Trust what feels most nourishing for you right now.

Anchored in Connection: The Power of Friendship and Partnership

There is also power in connecting with just one or two people at a time. Each week on Tuesday nights for the past 25 plus years, my closest friends, Jane and Jony (pictured here), jump on a three-way girls' call to dish on the latest happenings in our lives, including kids, jobs, spouses, health, future dreams, and other stuff that is too delicate to mention here. As we plowed through our graduate studies at UCLA, we became a best-friend trio.

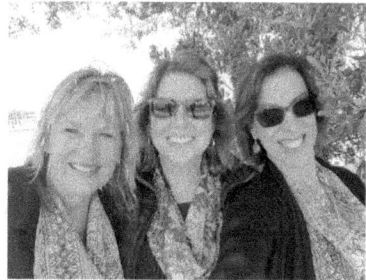

Friends like these gems are rare, brilliant, and hard to come by, so we hold on tight. We have been there for each other through boyfriends, weddings, kids, loss of loved ones, and a smorgasbord of health issues. Since they live in southern California and I live eight hours north, we make a point of meeting for a "gals' weekend" at least three times a year. Their wise counsel, mothering, coaching, cajoling, humor, support, funny noises, and inappropriate dance moves are woven into the very fabric of my being. Because of our deep trust, similar values, and long history, they are treasured members of my Board of Directors, guiding my company into the future. I am grateful for them every day, and I wouldn't have become the bold entrepreneur you know without their unwavering belief in me and constant encouragement to chase my dreams, even when the path felt uncertain.

Friendships are as meaningful as any other relationship in your life. Research and wisdom often suggest that having one to three close, deeply connected friends is enough to provide the emotional support, trust, and sense of belonging that enriches your life. Building friendships as an adult may take effort and vulnerability, but the connections you cultivate can be deeply fulfilling and enduring.

Alongside these treasured friendships, I am deeply grateful for the unwavering presence and love of my husband of 26 years, Kristapor. When we committed to marriage, he took a leap of faith. He chose love over tradition and stepped outside the expectations of his close-knit Armenian family to build a life with someone from a different background. His commitment to our partnership never wavered. With a solid belief that I was his person, he dove in with his whole heart. Two kids and more than two decades later, his family has fully welcomed me into their hearts.

Kris has created a deep sense of safety, allowing me to explore my true self, take professional leaps, and show up in the world more confidently. He is my anchor, cheering me on whether I'm launching a new course or working on dance choreography in our living room. As a hospital critical care pharmacist, he works tirelessly in a high-stakes environment, bringing compassion, calm, and clinical excellence to every shift. Around town, he's something of a local legend. When we go out to dinner, it's not unusual to hear someone call out, "Hey, KT!" followed by the glowing remark directed toward me, "Your husband is so smart." I smile, beaming with pride for the extraordinary man standing by my side.

Making Your Mental Health a Priority

As a healthcare professional, you may struggle to prioritize your mental health and well-being due to a combination of social, cultural, and personal pressures. It is ironic that in healthcare settings, there is often an unspoken expectation to "push through" and prioritize patient care over your personal needs.

How many times have you heard a colleague say they haven't gone to the bathroom since they started their shift, or they skipped lunch to plow through an overwhelming workload? You know the impact of this chronic stress and deprivation on our body and soul, but somehow, you have been programmed to carry on. Working overtime without complaint was the cultural norm when I worked at Stanford Hospital, and no one questioned those extra hours. It was just the way they did it there.

Many healthcare professionals feel guilty focusing on themselves when they perceive their patients' or job's needs as more urgent. Your identity may be tied to caregiving, and you might feel too embarrassed to focus on your own needs when you perceive others' needs as more pressing. This can lead to compassion fatigue, exacerbated by having to do double duty and caring for dependents or family members when you arrive home. You may also have your internal struggles or be a survivor of trauma. Whatever your situation, I hear and see you. My body had to wake me up with psychogenic seizures before I was willing to slow down and seek the mental health counseling I so desperately needed.

So, how can you preserve your well-being while serving others in your healthcare role? In addition to counseling, here are some simple actions you can take to maintain your best mental health.

Practice gratitude and reflection by taking time to notice and appreciate the joyous moments in your life. It could be the patient who acknowledged your care with a heartfelt squeeze of the hand or a coworker who brought you fresh oranges from their tree. This simple habit can help maintain a sense of purpose and balance, especially during stressful times. Keeping a gratitude journal or using an app to jot down things you're thankful for—even small wins or kind gestures—can help train your mind to focus on the good.

Practice kindness toward others regularly. Research shows that making kindness a habit uplifts those around us and improves our psychological and physical health. Whether writing a note of appreciation or hugging your partner for emptying the dishwasher, kindness boosts happiness on both ends. The person receiving kindness experiences joy, and the one giving it often feels even better.

Practice self-compassion. Dr. Kristin Neff, a pioneer in this field, reminds us, "Self-compassion is not about being self-indulgent or complacent; it's about realizing that you're worthy of love and care, even in your imperfections." This is especially vital for high-achieving healthcare professionals, who may have punishingly high internal expectations. Allow yourself a little grace, forgive your missteps, and take the rest you so often recommend to others.

Practice moments of awe to reconnect with a more profound sense of wonder and perspective. Awe invites us to step outside ourselves and feel part of something larger—whether learning a new concept, enjoying a piece of breathtaking music, or standing under a star-filled sky. These moments are inspiring and reduce stress, improve well-being, and shift how you see the world.

Spend time in nature to foster a connection with the earth and yourself. Nature provides a space for introspection, healing, and growth. Taking a walk in the fresh air, planting something in the soil, watching a hummingbird in flight, or simply listening to the rhythm of the ocean—these small moments in nature offer powerful medicine for the heart. These quiet observations can transform your mental health and nurture a deeper sense of resilience, joy, and inner peace.

Explore your creativity by giving yourself permission to take risks and create without judgment. Whether it's painting, dancing, cooking, writing, or playing music, the act of creating can be liberating and deeply fulfilling. The process matters more than the outcome; what's important is the space to express yourself freely and authentically.

Create space for Spiritual or Philosophical Reflection. Take time to connect with something greater than yourself. This could mean meditating, reading inspiring texts or quotes, journaling, or simply sitting in stillness. Carving out quiet moments for reflection helps ground you in meaning and clarity, especially in times of uncertainty.

Be Wildly Authentic and True to Yourself

One powerful way to begin living more authentically is by embracing this simple affirmation: "I give myself permission to be me." Authenticity has a ripple effect—it invites others to show up as themselves, too. When we dare to be real, we create space for others to take their own risks: to wear purple glasses, dance in public, dress like Superman, or read their poetry out loud. As Fred Rogers reminded us time and again on *Mister Rogers' Neighborhood,* "I like you just the way you are."

You may already be living from a place of authenticity; if not, that's okay. For many of us, it's a journey that unfolds over time. The beauty of choosing this path is that it allows you to show up fully as yourself with your strengths, quirks, vulnerabilities, and back story. You get to be you, beautiful you, without apology. At first, moving into a more authentic version of yourself may be scary and uncomfortable. To help out, look for role models who are already doing it. My friend Katy says her feelings kindly and without apology. "I don't want to do that," or "No, I don't agree." When I hesitate to speak my truth, I think of Katy, and then I state my truth. Nothing bad has happened to me yet. As a matter of fact, I feel more liberated.

As you continue paddling along your river of authenticity, you may find yourself more deeply connected to your mindbody and more attuned to your own needs and the people around you. You might notice you are more at ease with yourself and your colleagues at work. You might connect with patients more deeply and with less judgment. Your body may feel more grounded, your energy more aligned—like all eight cylinders are firing in sync. You might even open some doors to bidirectional healing in this space of presence and openness.

So, how do you get closer to your authentic self?

Here are a few practical ideas to explore. You don't need to try all these at once. Notice which one feels most relevant right now and start there.

As you experiment with something new, pay attention to how it affects you—physically, emotionally, even mentally. It might initially feel awkward or unfamiliar, but that's often just part of trying something different. Discomfort doesn't mean you're doing it wrong; it simply means you're moving in a new direction.

Spend time mind wandering and get to know yourself. Allow yourself quiet moments to connect with your feelings. Are you making time in your life for the things that are most important and healing for you? Check in with your mindbody and ask if it needs to tell you something or if it feels content and heard. On Saturday mornings, I leave my cell phone out of sight and give myself permission to walk outside, garden, declutter a shelf, organize my jewelry, or sit with a cup of tea and look out the window.

Express Your Truth. This is tricky since you don't want to make other people uncomfortable, but it is one of the most essential actions you can take to stand up for yourself. During a meeting with my Director of Operations, Bryanna bravely stated, "I am feeling anxious and overwhelmed with this project." At first, I felt bad that I might be causing her to feel this way since I assigned her the project. But then I realized that I was also feeling anxious and overwhelmed. For the past few days, I had been more scattered and less focused due to the complexity and challenges of this particular project. Hearing her state the truth about how she felt allowed me to acknowledge her feelings and recognize that I had similar thoughts.

Expressing the truth propelled us to create a new strategy to complete the project, which was less demanding and emotionally taxing. I thanked Bryanna for having the courage to share her feelings and let her know that it had allowed me to discover and express my emotions more authentically. Her simple statement also helped me realize that it's okay to say you feel overwhelmed and anxious. I used to think admitting those feelings was an indication of failure. Now, I see it in a new light. There is power and healing in expressing your feelings to those you feel safe with.

Are you willing to share your truth with someone you trust, to say your feelings out loud? The other person may feel the same way or pick up on your unspoken vibes. Take that risk and know that I am cheering you on!

Celebrate Your Uniqueness! I challenge you to recognize what makes you different and lean into it as a source of strength. Consider Temple Grandin, who is a PhD, professor, best-selling author, animal behaviorist, and autism self-advocate in top demand as an international speaker. As an individual with autism, Dr. Grandin describes her unique view of the world by saying, "I think in pictures." Unlike many people who process information through abstract concepts or words, her thoughts are like a series of vivid, detailed images, similar to a movie running in her mind. She leveraged her unique perspective to transform animal welfare and promote awareness of neurodiversity, inspiring and educating others through her pioneering work and advocacy.

Take some time to consider what makes you stand out from the crowd and start flaunting it! Ask your trusted friends and family if you are unsure what your secret sauce is. They will gladly help you recognize your gifts and encourage you to bring them to light.

Be Bold and Vulnerable. Authenticity requires courage to show the world your genuine self, even when it feels risky. After the pandemic, I felt a calling to teach a community belly dance class to bring people back together and celebrate the joy in life. Dancing creates a magical connection that transcends words. You can see the radiance in the faces of the students as they spin, shimmy, and move their bodies in new ways.

But I was struggling with a dilemma. I wasn't sure whether I was ready to dress up in a belly dance outfit and reveal my midriff while leading these dance classes. My abdominal muscles have been stretched from gestating two kids, and on the verge of 60, my belly has softened. Yet, the beauty of this dance form is that it welcomes all body types and encourages body positivity. I thought of brave actresses like Emma Thompson and Jamie Lee Curtis, who have courageously role-modeled how real women's bodies look, even if they're famous. I wanted to be bold and vulnerable like them, but an unwelcome inner voice tried to convince me that I should hide my belly. Getting ready for the first day of class, I pulled on my flowing skirt, wrapped my belly dance belt around my hips, and slipped into a sparkly purple cropped top. I tucked a flower in my hair, swiped on my brightest lipstick, looked in the mirror, and said, "Watch out, world. Here I come."

I opened the door, greeted each new dancer with a smile, and proudly demonstrated how to shake and shimmy what the good Lord gave me—belly and all. It was one of the best days of my life.

Bidirectional Healing - The Gift We Carry Forward

Writing this book began as a leap into the unknown and unfolded into something far greater than I ever imagined. Sharing this journey of discovery, joy, and resilience with you has been profoundly healing for me, and I hope it's offered moments of healing for you, too.

By entrusting you with my truth and lived experiences, I've freed a part of myself that had long remained hidden in the shadows. You, my wonderful healthcare colleagues, encouraged me to write this book.

And in doing so, you opened the door to your light of kindness. For that, I am forever grateful.

When we reclaim forgotten pieces of ourselves and find the courage to speak our truths, we reconnect with a deeper sense of meaning and possibility. In that space of renewed wholeness, something remarkable happens. Healing begins to flow both ways—between storyteller and listener, from caregiver to the one being cared for, and from parent to child. These moments of connection—vulnerable, honest, and human—allow us to experience bidirectional healing, which lies at the very heart of caregiving.

This is the healing gift we carry forward.

Final notes from Coach Beverly as you embrace the journey ahead

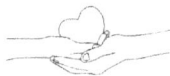

Take the risk. Say yes. Try that thing you've been putting off. Love your body exactly as it is. Be bold. Step into your authenticity. Make time to rediscover yourself. Think with your heart. Surrender. Show up. Move beyond your comfort zone and speak your truth. Get enough sleep. Ask for help when you need it. Stay connected to the people who lift you up. Seek out deep conversations, embrace your growth, and get ready for transformation.

I believe in you.

This is Coach Beverly, signing off.

EPILOGUE

When One Truth Makes Room for Another

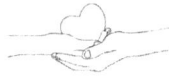

With this book on the verge of being published, I had to tell my mom that I was sharing in these pages what had lived unspoken between us for over five decades. After dinner on Mother's Day 2025, I recalled my childhood pain and how it shaped my life. My husband was present for support. The words kept pouring out of me, an unexpected flood of what I had so carefully concealed inside. I told her, "I felt an urgent need to write this book for my colleagues who might have also experienced trauma as children. I wanted them to know they weren't alone, and it wasn't their fault."

This moment between us was raw, uncomfortable, and scary. But my truth had been spoken. I finally felt like I could take a deep breath and release.

After a long pause, my mom shared her truth about what happened to her when she was five years old. A painful secret she had never shared with anyone. My husband hugged her and said, "It wasn't your fault," an offering of grace and forgiveness. And, in that exchange, I was able to see her not just as my mom but as a woman who had carried a lifetime of pain in silence.

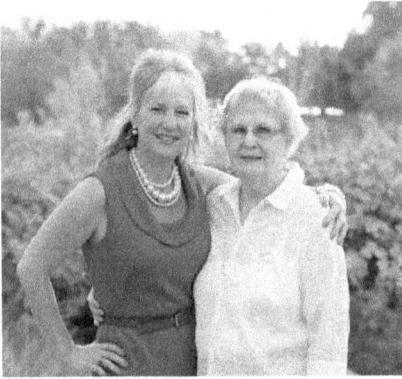

This exchange shifted something between us. It didn't erase the past but allowed space for compassion to disrupt the wall I had carefully constructed around my heart. As my mom and I navigate this uncharted journey forward, my hope is that we can create a renewed relationship built on honesty. One that acknowledges and allows space for our truest and messiest selves.

As I close this book, thank you for the work you do each day. For showing up for others, even when carrying your own pain. This book offers you permission to speak your truth. Permission to share your story. Permission to believe that healing, even if slow or imperfect, is possible when we are vulnerable. Sometimes, healing starts with being seen. And sometimes, telling your story helps someone else find the courage to tell theirs.

Reciprocity & Shared Purpose

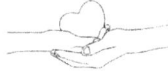

Mentoring the Next Generation of Diabetes Healthcare Professionals

Reciprocity honors the idea that when we give, we also receive, creating a continuous cycle of mutual benefit. Botanist and philosopher Robin Kimmerer, PhD, beautifully describes this as the covenant of reciprocity, a concept deeply rooted in Indigenous knowledge and ecological wisdom.

In this spirit, our company has made a ten-year commitment to mentor 500 healthcare professionals from diverse communities—empowering them to become Certified Diabetes Care and Education Specialists (CDCES) through our Bridge Program. But this initiative goes beyond certification. It's about cultivating relationships, expanding access, and building a thriving, inclusive community of diabetes care professionals.

The Bridge Program and Scholarship Fund are designed to foster equity in healthcare education by providing mentorship and financial support to professionals serving under-resourced communities. We are looking to partner with mentors and organizations who share this mission. A portion of all book proceeds will directly support our scholarship fund, extending the reach of this work even further.

Reciprocity builds and strengthens the bonds that hold communities together. When healthcare professionals feel seen, supported, and valued, they are more likely to extend that same compassion to the people they serve, creating healing and hope.

Lasting change is not the result of individual effort alone—it is born from mutual care and collective purpose. By embracing this cycle of giving and receiving, we uplift one another and create a legacy of transformation for future generations of healthcare professionals.

To learn more or get involved as a mentor or student in our Bridge Program, please visit www.DiabetesEd.net or email us at info@diabetesed.net.

Acknowledgments

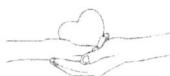

Writing Healing through Connection has been a journey of profound discovery, healing, and growth—one I could never have made alone. Translating the moments that shaped me into words proved more daunting than I ever imagined. Yet, this book kept knocking at my heart, insisting on being written, eager to leap onto these pages. I am deeply grateful to the many people who walked beside me along the way, cheering me over the finish line.

To my husband, Kris: Thank you for your thoughtful review of endless drafts and your steady listening as I wrestled through the content and message of this book. Your constant reminder to "think from your heart" is etched in my DNA. You are my anchor, cheerleader, and safe harbor.

To my boys: Robert, thank you for holding down the fort at DiabetesEd when I needed your help most. Jackson, thank you for being my sounding board and truth teller as I uncovered the deeper meaning of this book. I love you boys like crazy, and I am one proud mama.

To my besties, Jony and Jane: Your wisdom, humor, and fierce love are woven into every page of this book. Without your steadfast friendship, neither this book nor my company would exist in its current form. For over thirty years, you have lifted me up and gently nudged me forward, reminding me that I am enough.

To my mom: By courageously sharing your truth and allowing space for mine, you opened a door to healing for both of us.

To my Guilt-Free Book Club sisters, with a special shoutout to Dawn and Katy: Thank you for reading early drafts and offering valuable feedback that kept me pointed toward my true north. All of your encouragement has given me the space to be vulnerable, authentic, and wildly honest.

To my ReBellyon Shimmy Sisters: Dancing with you wonderful women every Wednesday for over fifteen years has been pure joy; a twirling reminder to celebrate life and embrace the magic. Thank you for your friendship, sparkle, and laughter.

To Simon Golden, PhD, who cajoled me into writing this book: You kept me on track, asked the tough questions, and provided plenty of encouragement. Thank you for helping me find what I needed to say.

To my editor, Kate Williams: You wrestled an explosion of ideas and paragraphs into a cohesive story. Your expert editing helped this book express its truest intention with verve and clarity.

To Bryanna and the Diabetes Education Services Team: I am truly honored to work alongside such intelligent, resilient, and compassionate individuals. Your unwavering dedication to building a platform that champions inclusive, person-centered diabetes education for healthcare professionals inspires me daily.

To Alex and Ying Chea: Thank you for believing in me long before I believed in myself. Inside the warm, busy walls of Ying's Kitchen, I learned some of life's most important lessons about hard work, generosity, and the beauty of everyday kindness. You are always with me.

To Lainey Koski, superwoman and my first business partner: You helped my company take flight and, along the way, you became a treasured friend who helped me believe anything was possible. Your spirit still hangs out with me in our office, providing gentle encouragement when I need it most.

To my dad: Thanks for making sure I knew how to hustle, question everything, and never let a fly ball slip past an open glove. I miss you.

To the healthcare professionals who inspire me every day: Thank you for reminding me, again and again, that connection is where true healing begins.

About the Author

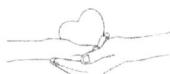

Beverly Thomassian, RN, MPH, CDCES, BC-ADM
The Compassionate Coach in Diabetes Care

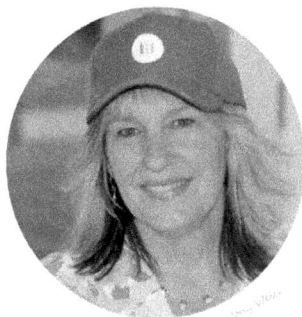

Coach Beverly is a nationally recognized diabetes nurse specialist, mentor, and author whose work bridges science, storytelling, and soul. With decades of experience, she is a passionate advocate for person-centered, inclusive care.

As founder of Diabetes Education Services™, Beverly has trained thousands of clinicians to achieve diabetes certification while championing a compassionate approach to healthcare. Whether dancing through moments of self-doubt or coaching professionals toward success, Beverly leads with authenticity and heart. Learn more by scanning the QR code below or visiting the author's website at www.diabetesed.net.

References

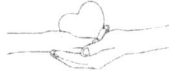

Chapter 1 Sources

Dube, S. R., Anda, R. F., Felitti, V. J., Chapman, D. P., Williamson, D. F., & Giles, W. H. (2001). Childhood abuse, household dysfunction, and the risk of attempted suicide throughout the life span: Findings from the Adverse Childhood Experiences Study. JAMA, 286(24), 3089–3096. https://doi.org/10.1001/jama.286.24.3089

ACEs Too High. (n.d.). Got your ACE score? https://acestoohigh.com/got-your-ace-score/

Parade, S. H., Huffhines, L., Daniels, T. E., Stroud, L. R., Nugent, N. R., & Tyrka, A. R. (2021). A systematic review of childhood maltreatment and DNA methylation: Candidate gene and epigenome-wide approaches. Translational Psychiatry, 11(1), 134. https://doi.org/10.1038/s41398-021-01207-y

Center for Substance Abuse Treatment (US). (2014). Understanding the impact of trauma. In Trauma-informed care in behavioral health services (Treatment Improvement Protocol (TIP) Series, No. 57). Substance Abuse and Mental Health Services Administration (US). https://www.ncbi.nlm.nih.gov/books/NBK207191/

Wing, R., Gjelsvik, A., Nocera, M., & McQuaid, E. L. (2015). Association between adverse childhood experiences in the home and pediatric asthma. Annals of Allergy, Asthma & Immunology, 114(5), 379–384. https://doi.org/10.1016/j.anai.2015.02.019

ACES Aware. (n.d.). Aces Aware. https://www.acesaware.org/

Adverse Childhood Experience Questionnaire for Adults
California Surgeon General's Clinical Advisory Committee

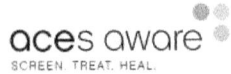

aces aware
SCREEN. TREAT. HEAL.

Our relationships and experiences—even those in childhood—can affect our health and well-being. Difficult childhood experiences are very common. Please tell us whether you have had any of the experiences listed below, as they may be affecting your health today or may affect your health in the future. This information will help you and your provider better understand how to work together to support your health and well-being.

Instructions: Below is a list of 10 categories of Adverse Childhood Experiences (ACEs). From the list below, please add up the number of categories of ACEs you experienced prior to your 18th birthday and put the total number at the bottom. (You do not need to indicate which categories apply to you, only the total number of categories that apply.)

1. Did you feel that you didn't have enough to eat, had to wear dirty clothes, or had no one to protect or take care of you?

2. Did you lose a parent through divorce, abandonment, death, or other reason?

3. Did you live with anyone who was depressed, mentally ill, or attempted suicide?

4. Did you live with anyone who had a problem with drinking or using drugs, including prescription drugs?

5. Did your parents or adults in your home ever hit, punch, beat, or threaten to harm each other?

6. Did you live with anyone who went to jail or prison?

7. Did a parent or adult in your home ever swear at you, insult you, or put you down?

8. Did a parent or adult in your home ever hit, beat, kick, or physically hurt you in any way?

9. Did you feel that no one in your family loved you or thought you were special?

10. Did you experience unwanted sexual contact (such as fondling or oral/anal/vaginal intercourse/penetration)?

Your ACE score is the total number of yes responses.

Do you believe that these experiences have affected your health?   ◯ Not Much   ◯ Some   ◯ A Lot

From www.AcesAware.org

Chapter 2 Sources

The Paper Crane. (1989). The American Journal of Nursing, 89(6), 824–825. Lippincott Williams & Wilkins. http://www.jstor.org/stable/3470798

Werner, D., Thuman, C., & Maxwell, J. (2009). Where there is no doctor: A village health care handbook. Hesperian Foundation. https://ia801902.us.archive.org/24/items/WhereThereIsNoDoctor-English-DavidWerner/14.DavidWerner-WhereThereIs-NoDoctor.pdf

Chapter 5 Sources

Abbott. (2025, February 4). Abbott's Above the Bias film reveals misconceptions can impact diabetes care. https://abbott.mediaroom.com/2025-02-04-Abbotts-Above-the-Bias-Film-Reveals-Misconceptions-Can-Impact-Diabetes-Care

Hessler, D. M., Fisher, L., Guzman, S., Strycker, L., Polonsky, W. H., Ahmann, A., Aleppo, G., Argento, N. B., Henske, J., Kim, S., Stephens, E., Greenberg, K., & Masharani, U. (2024). EMBARK: A randomized, controlled trial comparing three approaches to reducing diabetes distress and improving HbA1c in adults with type 1 diabetes. Diabetes Care, 47(8), 1370–1378. https://doi.org/10.2337/dc23-2452

Dickinson, J. K., Guzman, S. J., Maryniuk, M. D., O'Brian, C. A., Kadohiro, J. K., Jackson, R. A., D'Hondt, N., Montgomery, B., Close, K. L., & Funnell, M. M. (2017). The use of language in diabetes care and education. Diabetes Care, 40(12), 1790–1799. https://doi.org/10.2337/dci17-0041

Chapter 6 Sources

Tomasovic, L. (2024, January 10). Beyond the Renaissance: Nobel laureates and their creative pursuits. Perspectives in Research – Johns Hopkins Medicine. https://biomedicalodyssey.blogs. hopkinsmedicine.org/2024/01/beyond-the-renaissance-nobel-laureates-and-their-creative-pursuits/

Teixeira-Machado, L., Arida, R. M., & Mari, J. J. (2019). Dance for neuroplasticity: A descriptive systematic review. Neuroscience & Biobehavioral Reviews, 96, 232–240. https://doi.org/10.1016/j.neubiorev.2018.12.010

Herold, F., Hamacher, D., Schega, L., & Müller, N. G. (2018). Thinking while moving or moving while thinking—Concepts of motor-cognitive training for cognitive performance enhancement. Frontiers in Aging Neuroscience, 10, 228. https://doi.org/10.3389/fnagi.2018.00228

Chapter 8 Sources

Siegel, J. S., Subramanian, S., Perry, D., et al. (2024). Psilocybin desynchronizes the human brain. Nature, 632, 131–138. https://doi.org/10.1038/s41586-024-07624-5

Murthy, V. H. (2020). Together: Why social connection holds the key to better health, higher performance, and greater happiness. Harper Wave.

Sheehan, C. M., Frochen, S. E., Walsemann, K. M., & Ailshire, J. A. (2019). Are U.S. adults reporting less sleep?: Findings from sleep duration trends in the National Health Interview Survey, 2004–2017. Sleep, 42(2), zsy221. https://doi.org/10.1093/sleep/zsy221

Other Books Mentioned

Cameron, J. (2002). The artist's way: A spiritual path to higher creativity. Tarcher/Putnam. (Original work published 1992)

Gilbert, E. (2015). Big magic: Creative living beyond fear. Riverhead Books.

Maté, G., & Maté, D. (2022). The myth of normal: Trauma, illness, and healing in a toxic culture. Avery.

Neff, K. (2011). Self-compassion: The proven power of being kind to yourself. William Morrow.

Oliver, M. (1986). Dream work. Atlantic Monthly Press.

Perry, B. D., & Winfrey, O. (2021). What happened to you? Conversations on trauma, resilience, and healing. Flatiron Books.

Strayed, C. (2015). Brave enough. Alfred A. Knopf.

Van der Kolk, B. A. (2014). The body keeps the score: Brain, mind, and body in the healing of trauma. Viking.

Bring energy, expertise, and inspiration to your next event with Coach Beverly

Beverly Thomassian, RN, MPH, CDCES, BC-ADM, brings decades of clinical expertise, heartfelt storytelling, and a passion for human-centered care to every presentation. Beverly offers keynote talks on her groundbreaking book *Healing through Connection*, exploring how presence, empathy, and authenticity can transform the healthcare experience and support professional well-being.

She also provides a variety of evidence-based presentations on diabetes management, emerging therapies, ADA Standards of Care, and person-centered care approaches. Attendees leave with powerful insights on building meaningful connections with those they serve, their teams, and themselves. To book Coach Beverly for your event, visit www.DiabetesEd.net or email info@diabetesed.net. You can also call us at 530/ 592-5943.

Ready to launch your career in diabetes education or renew your certification? Visit our website for expert courses, free resources, and the support you need to succeed!

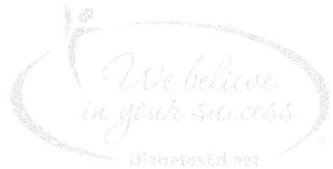

If you're interested in entering the rewarding field of diabetes education or pursuing your diabetes certification, our website is your go-to resource. At Diabetes Education Services, we offer expert-led courses, free webinars, practice tests, and supportive tools to help you gain the confidence and knowledge needed to succeed. Whether you're just starting your journey or a seasoned professional, we offer courses for every stage of your career at DiabetesEd.net.

FREE Clinical Resources at www.DiabetesEd.net

Sign up for our **monthly newsletter** to stay connected with your diabetes education community and the latest news, updates, and resources to support your journey toward excellence in care.

Medication and Insulin PocketCards - Our diabetes medication cards summarize the action, dosing, and considerations for today's available diabetes drugs.

Enjoy our **Resource Library**, which includes webinars on certification, the CDCES Coach App, Cheat Sheets that summarize standards, medications, recommended apps, and much more.

www.ingramcontent.com/pod-product-compliance
Lightning Source LLC
Chambersburg PA
CBHW060854280326
41934CB00007B/1043